DANCE AS A HEALING ART

Returning to Health with Movement & Imagery

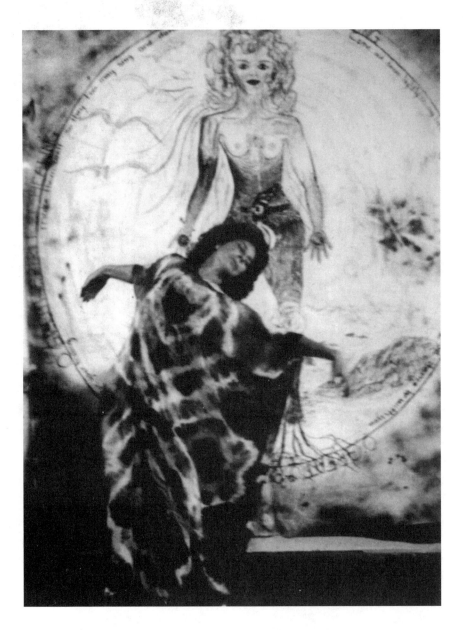

I imagine my breath as water flowing through my body,

cleansing and healing me from cancer.

ANNA HALPRIN, 1975

Mom —
you were born to
move your body, and
you know it ♡ Gigi

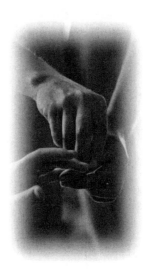

DANCE AS A HEALING ART

Returning to Health with Movement & Imagery

BY ANNA HALPRIN

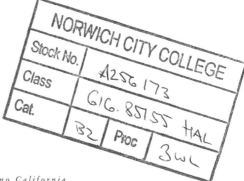
EDITED & PUBLISHED BY SIEGMAR GERKEN, Ph.D.

LifeRhythm Books of Mendocino California

C O P Y R I G H T

Produced in the LifeRhythm Energy Field

Editors: Rachel Kaplan and Siegmar Gerken
Cover and Layout Design: Elizabeth Ives Manwaring
Proofreader: Elinor Lindheimer
Coordinators: Dixie Black Shipp, Susan Wells and Debra Dizin

Library of Congress Cataloging-in-Publication Data

Halprin, Anna
   Dance as a healing art: returning to health through movement and imagery/Anna Halprin.
      296 p.
      Includes bibliographical references
      ISBN 0-940795-19-1
      1. Dance therapy. I Title
      2.
RM931.D35 H34 2000
616.8'5155—de21

©LifeRhythm 2000
Post Office Box 806
Mendocino CA 95460
Telephone: 707.937.1825
Facsimile: 707.937.3052
Books@LifeRhythm.com

ISBN# 0-940795-19-1

PRINTED ON ACID FREE PAPER

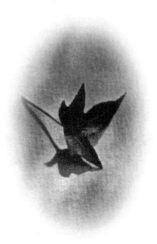

DEDICATION

TO ALL THOSE LIVING WITH CANCER AND THEIR LOVED ONES

WHO HAVE LEARNED TO COPE WITH THEIR FEAR,

ENDURE THEIR PAIN, AND FIND THE

COURAGE TO CONTINUE.

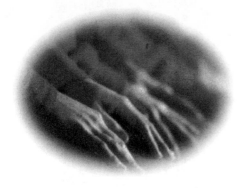

TABLE OF CONTENTS

This book is not intended as a substitute for competent medical treatment.
Its intention is to support the process of healing in all creative ways.

A C K N O W L E D G E M E N T S

I owe thanks for this book to:

The Lloyd Symington Foundation, which commissioned it,

The Tamalpa Institute, which insisted on it,

Maggie Creighton and the Cancer Support Center, who initiated it,

Peggy Rogers, who nourished it,

Mike Samuels, who contributed to it,

Rachel Kaplan, who edited it,

Elizabeth Ives Manwaring, who designed it,

And Siegmar Gerken, who did the final editing and published it.

The first time I met Anna Halprin was in 1987, one week after my mastectomy, in a group with other cancer patients at the Cancer Support and Education Center in Menlo Park, California. We were there to fight for our lives without the least notion of what that meant or how to do it. We were a diverse group: two nuns, two divorced women (one with grown children, one with young children and metastasized cancer), three couples ranging in age from their 30s to 60s, a gay man, and a 19-year-old woman with Hodgkin's Lymphoma. We were ordinary people in extraordinary circumstances. We were all following conventional treatments, hoping they would eliminate the cancer. Yet we were also sitting in this group, as part of a program that told us we could have an effect on our own healing.

Maybe we all came hoping the program would be like a doctor's visit, that Maggie Creighton, Anna Halprin, and the other facilitators had the answer. We would receive their wisdom, like a pill, and we would be healed. But it wasn't like that. From the beginning, it was clear that to do this work, we would have to access our bodies' healing ability and communicate between our conscious desire to live and some unconscious, seemingly automatic internal process. This would be a journey, an expedition into unknown territory, and Anna and Maggie would be our guides.

The trick was, they didn't know our paths. They had been to the jungle before, but each new trip is like plunging into uncharted territory. There are no road maps. The wonderful thing about Anna is that she is a master guide, a tracker of the soul, willing to take these expeditions with us. As a dancer, schooled in form, she could have come up with exercises, or a set of movements to unlock our energy. But Anna saw healing as a journey into our own inner being; her goal was to unlock our personal knowledge, the rhythm and movement inside each of us. When I took my own journey, I found I had to be quite brave. It was as exciting, and as fraught with danger, as any new world explorer has ever encountered. I am grateful to have had Anna as one of my guides.

I have since gone on to be a guide for others who, like myself, come to this work to fight for their lives. I have to resist the temptation to tell them what I did, or what they should or should not do. I can't tell them what image to use for their healing, or what treatment to take, or that even if they follow their own intuition they will be cured. The more I work in this field, the more I respect each person's journey. There is no "cure" for cancer, or the myriad immune-suppressed conditions that are now prevalent. The most I can do is travel with a person, offer them a paddle when appropriate, show them how to use it, share with them my resources, listen to them, hold them, honor their courage, wisdom, and differences, and support them as they try to make sense of their experience.

To become an explorer is to leave one's comfort zone. It means leaving our familiar surroundings and entering places not yet known to us. To explore ourselves and our healing, to take this journey of the senses through our illness and to bring new meaning into our lives through this journey, is to visit those parts of our experience that have been hidden in darkness, like the jungle, or the ocean depths, or a rapidly flowing river. To choose to become an explorer is to choose to move forward instead of clinging to the rocks, to see where we are going and learn new skills that enable us to run the rapids. I have had the privilege to work with Anna in these dangerous territories for over nine years. I have watched her work grow and change. I have watched when she comes to visit my groups, and do a special session with them. I know these people before Anna arrives, and then I work with them after she has gone. Anna's process is so fluid that people are able to use it in many ways. Her work is like a fine dance between our unrecognized needs, our body wisdom, and our resistance. Sometimes people repeat our workshop and I have an opportunity to see change over time. I can see then how Anna's work is not about dying, it is about accessing our inner strength and desires, which are important for our living.

Anna has a unique ability to take her talents, her skills, and her personal experiences, use them to grow, and then help others do the same. Here is a woman who is a dancer. Here is a woman who takes dance into a community context, involving people in the creation of their own healing dances. Here is a woman who had a direct experience of drawing something unexplainable, unknown in her body. Here is a woman who chose to listen and make sense of that drawing, trusting that her body knew something her mind did not know. Here is woman who diagnosed her own cancer through her senses. Here is a woman who chose to use her senses to heal. Here is a woman who drew her dark side, that which is unexplored, and who moved that dark side, becoming the explorer. Here is a woman whose cancer disappeared. Here is a woman who has transformed that experience into a process for us all to use. This is the beauty of Anna's work.

Ultimately, it is not just about using our senses to cure an illness. This work is about learning to use our senses to expand and increase our intimacy with ourselves and thus improve the quality of our lives. But we don't know how to do that directly and so we have mediators, allies, forms, images, dances. These are the road maps Anna has developed over the years, and she pulls them out of her pack, like a compass, or a trusted tent, and shares them with us. As we play with these images and movements, they become more familiar and comfortable to us. We can begin to imagine using our energy in these ways in our daily life; and we begin to enrich our lives because the jungle suddenly isn't so dark or so tangled. Where we could only crawl before, now we can soar.

PEGGY ROGERS, M.A., MFCC

Director of Client Services, Cancer Support & Education Center

Menlo Park, California March, 1997

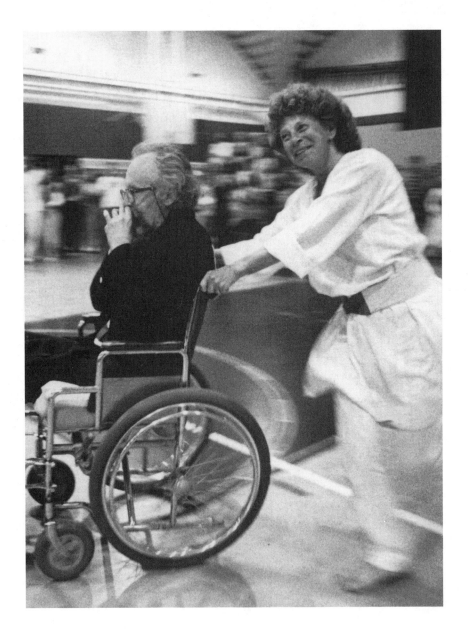

Anna Halprin dances with a man playing the harmonica.

As I continued teaching, it became apparent that the experience of movement connected to feelings generates long-buried and unknown emotions and images. When these emotions and images are expressed through movement, we dance. And when these dances are connected to our lives, they bring about dramatic release and change in our will to live. — ANNA HALPRIN

BRIEF HISTORY

I was born in Winnetka, Illinois in 1920. I have danced for as long as I can remember, and I have also had cancer and survived. So in 1980, when my friend and former student Maggie Creighton asked me to join her staff at the Cancer Support and Education Center in Menlo Park, California to offer a movement and dance session for people living with cancer, I did not hesitate to say yes. Turning to dance as a healing art had helped me, and healed me, and taught me some of the greatest lessons of my life. I remembered my own struggle with cancer and was happy to have a chance to share what I had learned with other people experiencing the same illness.

Dance as a healing art is traditional in many non-Western cultures, but this application of dance has been obscured and ignored in the Western world. I think this is a great loss and I believe we must reclaim what has been forgotten as we learn more about healing, illness, and death. When Maggie asked me to teach at her center, I embarked on this quest of reclamation. At that time, I didn't know why dance healed, I only knew that it did. The ways I had used dance in my own healing process were derived from a largely intuitive source, so I knew that if I wanted this work to be useful to others, I would have to find simple and direct road maps to lead the way. This book is about some of the maps I have discovered so far, and how I have applied them in practice.

The Cancer Support and Education Center's approach to healing cancer is to engage the whole person by emphasizing psychotherapeutic techniques, guided imagery, meditation, and other mind/body-based therapies. In keeping with this approach to the body, in my workshops I introduced sensory awareness exercises, and expressive movement and dance to the people at the Center. I knew from their first responses that this approach enabled us to go deeply, to a level beyond and below words. Insights into primary life issues and illness were revealed through dance in profound and unique ways that stretched past rational thought. And despite the difficulty of people's circumstances, we had fun! Participants were able to laugh as well as cry. They were pleased with their creativity, and quickly understood that movement and dance was accessible to them. In addition, they felt better and their life force was heightened. These early sessions encouraged me to continue exploring the healing power of dance. I very much wanted to reclaim this forgotten art and explore its enormous possibilities.

MOVING TOWARD LIFE

While still teaching at the Cancer Center, I furthered my explorations of dance as a healing art in a series of ongoing classes sponsored by the Tamalpa Institute. The Tamalpa Institute, co-founded by myself and Daria Halprin-Khalighi, is a center for expressive arts education. Beginning in 1986 and continuing up to the present time, Tamalpa has been sponsoring a program called Moving Toward Life for people living with cancer, their caregivers, and health professionals in the field. These classes are accessible to men and women of all backgrounds and economic status. No one is turned away for any reason and over 500 people from all walks of life have taken part in these programs. The results have been inspiring. There is a very high record of cancer survivors and people in remission among the people who have taken the class.

I do not claim that dance can cure a person with cancer, but through these classes, I have seen that dance has the power to heal. Healing is intrinsic to one's outlook on life. Someone with a strong will to live, someone who is willing to believe in the power of dance, someone who is determined and will not give up has a better chance of surviving cancer than someone who blindly follows the advice of her doctors and does not participate in her own healing. People who take an active role in relationship to their doctors, who consider many factors, including diet, prayer, existing complementary thera-pies, and lifestyle itself, have a better rate of survival. People who survive cancer often have a creative and holistic approach to living, and a sense of adventure. I have found it very stimulating and inspiring to teach people who have this attitude.

DANCE AS AN INTEGRATIVE THERAPY

There is a distinction between "curing" and "healing," which is useful when we approach dance, or any of the arts, as a healing modality. To "cure" is to physically elim-inate a disease. In the case of cancer, this is usually done through surgery, chemothera-py, radiation, or other treatments aimed at the physical body. To "heal" is to operate on many dimensions simultaneously, by aiming at attaining a state of emotional, mental, spiritual, and physical health. Healing also addresses the psychological dimension and works with belief systems, whether they are life-enhancing or destructive. It is possible, therefore, that a person with a terminal diagnosis may not be cured, but can be healed, and inversely, that someone can be cured, but not healed. Taken together, the healing process and the curative efforts of standard medicine support both the expansion and extension of life.

It is, of course, our greatest ideal to be both cured and healed. I recall how, after my operation for cancer, my doctor said to me, "You're just fine now. You are cured of can-cer. You can live a normal life as before," and I answered him by saying, "That's funny because I don't feel just fine. I'm scared. I don't know why I was stricken with cancer, or what kind of life I can live right now." I had been cured, perhaps, but not healed. For this reason, I personally encourage people to follow an integrated approach to health that is inclusive of Western and so-called "alternative" medicine. I am very careful to make no claim that the work described in this book should be used as one's sole treat-ment for cancer, or even that it extends life. I am certain, on the other hand, that it does expand or transform the quality of life. There is also intriguing evidence that in some cases, people who undertake healing processes that make sense to them can extend their lives as well as expand them.

In the 1970s, Carl O. Simonton, M.D., and Stephanie Matthews-Simonton, psychotherapist, pioneered the use of visualizations with meditation and therapeutic techniques in their treatment of people with terminal cancer. In 1975, this approach to the mind/body connection was not taken seriously. The idea that visualizations could affect the course of an illness was considered ridiculous. Since then, additional research has more than substantiated the validity of their pioneering work. Dr. David Spiegel did a research study in the 1980s at Stanford University that has done much to prove the importance of the mind/body connection to illness. He wanted to disprove the theory that there was a connection between psychotherapy and health, and was amazed instead to find a definite and convincing correlation. His study showed that cancer patients who joined a support group as a adjunct to their medical treatment doubled their survival time.

Dr. Spiegel's study, coming from within the established medical profession, gave credibility to the important link between the way our attitudes and emotions influence our health, an idea I had been exploring through dance since the early 1970s. The acceptance of expressive arts therapy, and dance in particular, as a healing modality is gaining momentum. On December 5, 1996, the *San Francisco Chronicle* carried an article on new directions in the medical scene stating, "Dr. Laura Esserman, a surgeon and co-director of the University of California, San Francisco Breast Care Center, is planning to lead an 'integrated approach' to breast cancer treatment that mixes conventional treatments such as surgery, chemotherapy and radiation with meditation, yoga, dance and art therapies." *(Emphasis mine)*. This is progress, indeed.

I had been using a combination of drawing images, writing about them, and dancing them with children since 1945 as a method for generating creativity in my children's dance classes. I found the process so intriguing that I began to use it with adults. In 1972, I did a drawing of myself in one of my classes and drew a round gray mass in my pelvic region. Partly because I resisted dancing this image, it struck me that there might be something wrong. It turned out that I had drawn my own malignant tumor. I had an operation and three years later a recurrence. This time, I drew a self-portrait to heal myself and I danced the drawing. Afterwards, I went into spontaneous remission. This may sound strange and unbelievable, but in recent years more and more doctors and therapists acknowledge this phenomenon. The late Dr. Brendan O'Regan, who did his research through the Noetic Science Institute, reported 800 cases of spontaneous remission. It can and does happen; I do not believe anyone knows exactly how.

The new acceptance of the mind/body connection in the healing process builds a bridge between the fields of expressive arts therapy and Western medicine. This bodes well for an integration of both our intuitive and rational knowledge about healing. It is also a way for expressive arts therapies to become more widely accepted and used by people in this culture, who have mostly been conditioned to believe that the mind and body are separate entities which do not reflect upon one another. The history of cancer research reminds us to appreciate the immensity of what we have yet to learn about the impact of the mind/body connection on the course of illness. The next frontier is to begin to explore the impact of expressive arts therapies, especially dance, in the treatment of illness. Dance seems particularly important because it can engage all the arts: movement, drawing, writing, music, and drama. Dance has a highly integrative nature. Exploring this expressive art modality is a beginning step toward reclaiming the healing power of dance.

As a result of my experiences, the road maps I discovered have taken many new turns. This book represents what I have learned so far. I hope you will be inspired to work in your own way with these materials. I want to encourage you to always engage your own creativity and powers of perception in the creation of classes for people with cancer. I offer a road map to the territory but not the territory itself. To arrive there, you must remain alert to what is unfolding in front of you, and use all your resources to respond to that moment. I want to encourage you to remain sensitive to the central inquiry of this work: How can we create change? How can we use dance to facilitate our healing? How can we access the power of dance to heal? The following chapter will give you background in the basic components, and a theoretical basis of this approach to creative movement.

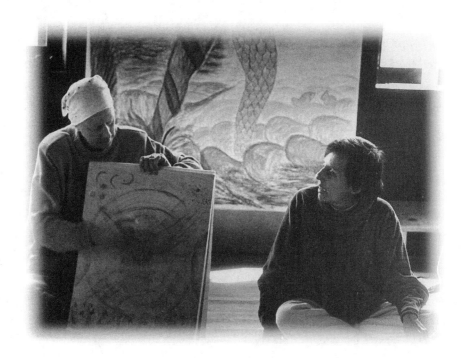

THE QUALITY OF SHARING IS

RESPECTFUL AND SUPPORTIVE.

When I first started working at the Cancer Center, I didn't know what to expect or how to specifically shape my material. I was encouraged by the responses I got to the movement exercises I presented, and I quickly began to research different ways of using the healing potential of dance. As I began to teach dance sessions in a number of venues, for varying lengths of time, and to different sorts of people at various stages of wellness, I noticed that in spite of the differences, a common thread ran through the classes. I was able to identify the four components I believe are intrinsic to this approach to movement, and which were included in each session I taught. These are the realms of sensation, movement, feelings/emotions, and imagery. Although material regarding all of these aspects will be presented separately in this book, it is important to remember that these components function continually in a mutual feedback process. They cannot, in truth, be separated. Movement affects the way we feel; the way we feel affects the way we move. This in turn feeds the images evoked. In working with dance, a holistic art form, our intention is to help the participant understand herself in an integrated manner.

D E F I N I N G   T E R M S

Throughout this book, I make a distinction between the words "sensing," "feeling," and "emotion." The dictionary gives a broad definition of "sensation," including "sentiment, emotion and passion." It also refers to sensation as a way to think of feeling. You might say "feel" this and mean "touch" this. The interchange of these words can be confusing. For our purposes, I would like to define the words as follows:

"*S e n s i n g*" refers to the physical sensations of the body.

For example, you might ask questions like these to help people bring awareness to their bodies: What do you sense at this moment? Do you sense any tightness anywhere? Do you sense heat or cold in any part of your body? Do you sense your eyelids trembling when you close them? Do you sense your shoulders lifting? Do you sense the difference when you let go and drop them?

"*Feelings*" refers to moods, such as grumpy , romantic, upset, impatient, or vulnerable.

"*Emotions*" rest behind "*Feelings.*"

They are deeper layers of feelings, such as love, hate, fear, grief, ecstasy, etc. They are the deepest responses we have to our life experiences.

LIFE / ART PROCESS

A direct type of movement that anyone can do is the basis of this approach. Therefore, the material in each class is accessible to everyone. A larger purpose of this work is to use simple movements that will generate immediate and personal responses. This direct approach to movement enables each person to connect to her own creative experience, rather than trying to imitate someone else's. It is the purpose of this work to integrate physical movement with feelings, emotions, personal images, and spirit. It is, in essence, a holistic approach.

When our dances are connected to our real-life issues in this manner, it is called the Life/Art Process. This method of working with dance seeks to access the life story of each person, and then use this life story as the ground for creating art. This is based upon the principle that *as life experience deepens, personal art expression expands, and as art expression expands, life experiences deepen.* I have found this interactive process to be especially effective when applied to people living with cancer. This book is about a way that everyone can discover a healing dance of their own though this Life/Art Process.

SENSATIONS

Dance is a medium of the body and our instrument of expression. It helps us become present in many ways. Our first step with this work is to enter and inhabit our bodies. We do this through our senses. Our sensations are the pathway leading us into the body.

Before you read further, make a list of the senses.

They are: <u>sight, sound, touch, smell, and taste.</u> There are <u>also motor and kinesthetic</u> senses. Invariably people tend to forget these last two. Did you remember them? If you did, you are the exception. Most people do not, although the kinesthetic and motor senses occupy the largest part of our brains. Perhaps we forget this because these senses have been dulled by the way most of us live. Our lives are dominated by sitting in cars and driving, sitting and watching TV, sitting and working at desks or drafting boards. Sitting, sitting, sitting... When we walk, it is usually on cement. We wear confining shoes for protection and lose the touch of the earth and the sensations of our feet. In urban centers we must protect ourselves by shutting out the overload of the noise and smells that surround us.

Almost everything in our modern industrialized society denies the life of the body and rewards the life of the mind. Fritz Perls, innovator of <u>Gestalt therapy,</u> had this well-known saying: "<u>Lose your head and come to your senses</u>." Our usual response to the over-stimulation in our lives is to tune out our senses. When we do this, we leave our bodies and in a way, we leave home, set adrift from the rich world within us. This inner world houses our feelings, our emotions, and our spirit. It holds the memories of our ancestors, our past, our present, and our future. Each of us lives in a body that has taken millions of years to evolve and which will continue to evolve as we pass from one generation to the next. Each of us has a unique body; there is not another one like it anywhere in the universe. And <u>this body is intricately designed to survive. It has wisdom, wonder, and magic in it to perform the great dance of life.</u> Our personal and cultural abandonment of our bodies can create illness, and a void in understanding how to regain our health. When we become ill, we may feel that our body, which we have taken for granted, has suddenly betrayed us. At this time, it is crucial to return to our bodies, to return home and reawaken our senses, so that the natural healer within can renew its strength and power.

Take a moment to open your ears and listen to the sounds around you. What do you hear? Then, look around you with fresh eyes as if seeing for the first time. What do you see? Smell a bay leaf, touch the rough bark of a tree, go for a blindfold walk in the woods, walk outside in the light of a full moon, roll in the warm sand or the cold snow,

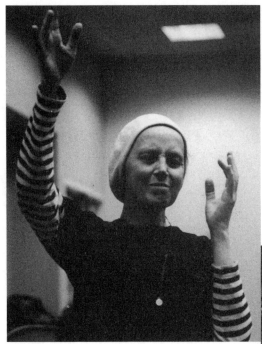

"Please let people in the group
know I am doing well."

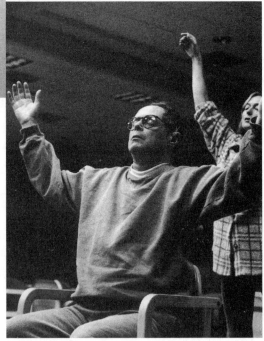

"My hands are an act of loving."

go for a plunge in the ocean, grow a garden and get your hands in the dirt, take your shoes and stockings off and walk barefoot in the grass. The next time it rains, take your clothes off and let it rain down on your naked body. Be wild, have fun, enjoy your sensations; inhabit your body and all its wonder. This is something children know how to do, and something adults have often forgotten.

The other day after a heavy rain I was taking a walk and passed a little girl who was stomping her feet wildly in a puddle of water. She was giggling as the water splashed all around her. She wore bright red shiny boots that made a clapping sound as they hit the water and her whole body was filled with joy. Her smiling parents stood patiently waiting until their little girl had finished her stomping water dance and then they all walked on, their pace a little brighter.

M O V E M E N T

When you think of dance and movement do you think of ballet, a modern or jazz dance, or some other form of stylized movement? Many people are shy about dance because of this association. This is not the way I think of dance movement at all. Dance can be approached as a direct and natural way to move without any personalized aesthetics imposed from an outside authority. Dance is not necessarily graceful, pretty, or spectacular. Dance can be grotesque, ugly, clumsy, funny, frightening, and conflicted. It can stomp, fall, attack, clutch, and reach. It can open, close, tip-toe, crawl, twist, turn, pound, jump, run, or skip. We can move together, or alone. We can move backwards, sideways, up and down. Movement is happening everywhere all the time. It is the motion of our cells, the pulse of our blood, the rhythm of our breath. It is, as well, the ocean waves rising and falling and the alternating patterns of night and day. Movement is life and movement is the source of dance. Any body, no matter how old or young, in whatever physical condition, has a capacity to move, even if it is just your little finger or a movement carried as an image in your mind's eye.

A woman in the advanced stages of cancer shared an experience in class which illustrates this point. She said she had just gotten an audio tape I sent her of guided movements. She wanted to follow it but felt unable to move because she was so weak. She told us she put it on anyway, and just moved her eyes and her hands. She had a deep experience. I know a man who was in a brutal automobile accident and lay in a hospital bed for months in a cast up to his neck. A healer came to visit him every day and guided him through imaginary kinesthetic activities, such as walking along the beach, or riding a bicycle. In his mind, he went hiking and swimming. He rode a horse and played tennis. They did this for months. In defiance of his doctor's prediction that he would not walk again, when the cast was removed he threw his legs over the side of the bed, stood up, unsteady but determined, and he walked. Movement can exist in the mind's eye and have a powerful effect. No matter what physical condition a person is in, it is important to remember that there is still a possible connection to movement.

THE FEEDBACK PROCESS BETWEEN MOVEMENT AND FEELINGS

When movement is liberated from the constricting armor of stylized, pre-conceived gestures, an innate feedback process between movement and feelings is generated. For example, try throwing your arms into the air above your head with vigor and say out loud, "I'm so depressed." Now cross your arms over your chest and double over, saying, "I feel so happy." The movement and the emotional feedback between these two things is so incongruous that it seems absurd. Throwing your arms in the air is uplifting. It can inspire a feeling of victory and celebration. Doubling over is more congruent to pain or fear.

This feedback process between movement and feelings is an essential ingredient of expressive movement. When you understand this, movement becomes a vehicle for releasing feelings which are essential in the healing process. Repressed or incongruent emotions shut down the immune system, causing pain and illness. We are working toward expression and congruency, and understanding movement and feelings in a constantly circulating feedback loop facilitates this process.

Keeping in mind the connection between movements and feelings, you will need to expose participants to a variety of movement qualities because they will then give rise to a variety of emotional responses. Flowing, jerky, strong, soft, expansive, contracted, reaching, retreating, fast, and slow movements are but a few examples of movement qualities. Each one will arouse a different feeling or emotional response. It is important to explore as many of them as you can. A particular movement may reveal a feeling or emotion never experienced before by a participant. It might reveal itself as an important aspect in someone's personal story which needs to be expressed and heard. Since there are infinite ways to move, we have the wonderful possibility of experiencing an infinite number of feelings and emotions.

Sometimes we may block ourselves from certain movements because unconsciously we are afraid of the feelings that will arise. For example, I have seen strong women go limp when asked to execute a forceful beating or kicking movement. This is usually because they are afraid to experience their anger. I have seen men experience soft, flowing, and lyrical movements which trigger off new and exciting feelings for them. One of the greatest values in working with the feedback process between movement and feelings is that it allows us to explore a wider range of movement qualities. Once we are able to experience an unfamiliar movement, it will often provide us with new emotional resources.

We each have our blind spots when it comes to how we move, and these same blind spots are apt to exist in the way we live our lives. For example, one woman in class discovered, after some hesitation, that she could move with force and strength even though it was difficult at first. She came back the next week and reported that when she was driving in the car with her partner, she began to feel anger welling up. For the very first time in her life she was able to express it without fear. She was amazed that this was acceptable, and that she felt so good. Since so much of our ability to experience and express ourselves fully lies in this relationship between movement and feelings, as teachers we need to be careful to offer a broad spectrum of movement possibilities. Remember that it works the other way as well: as we develop a broad vocabulary of movement, we have greater freedom to express the way we feel.

FEELINGS AND EMOTIONS

It is important to keep in mind that in this work, movement is the key player. Our feelings and emotions are channeled into movement. It is vital that the participants have a safe place to express their own experience, be it fear, envy, tenderness, love, sexuality, or passion. It does not matter. All judgment and moralistic behavior is suspended. Here is an example of emotions being channeled into movement. One day when we began class, a woman began to talk very fast, and in between sobs, she became hysterical, and somewhat incoherent. I asked her to shift from verbalizing and to start moving how she was feeling. She began dancing her feelings, which shifted gradually into another state. As she stopped speaking and began moving, I noticed she was holding her breath. "Breathe," I said, and every time anyone else in the group noticed something strained in her body, they would give her a signal to pay attention to it. In a few minutes, she had calmed herself. Her tears turned to a smile. This came to her by shifting her emotional expression to a movement expression. She was not guided to cut off her feelings, but rather, to go deeper into them through movement; this helped her find release and move on to the next phase in her process.

I M A G E R Y

"One of the things about people who are sick is that they have no control of physical reality. Their body is changing without them doing it. So taking a blank piece of paper and putting the image down is the first step towards controlling the rest of their life. They are controlling the outer-world." — M I K E   S A M U E L S

The feedback process between movement, feelings, and images operates on a level below words. It is not always possible to understand the content of what we feel, where our feelings come from, or how to apply the feelings that arise to our personal lives. In trying to understand the messages our body is giving us, rather than analyzing or interpreting in a cognitive way, participants make drawings of the images in their mind's eye in response to their movements and feelings. When we draw these images on paper or canvas, they are called visualizations. When we connect these image to our movements and feelings/emotions through dance, I call them Psychokinetic Visualizations.

CONFRONTATION
"You're not good enough."

VISUALIZATION
Visualizations depicting four stages of healing.

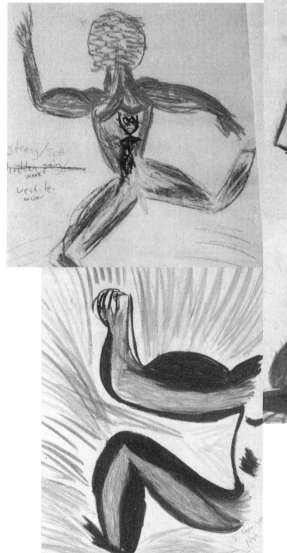

CHANGE
"5 days later at the end of the workshop, a second self-portrait."

RELEASE
"I fear you not."

The Psychokinetic Visualization Process has three parts. We go inside to find our personal image; we draw it on a piece of paper; and then we take this image into movement, we "dance" it. When doing this process, participants draw on a piece of paper that is 18" by 22," big enough for them to draw freely, but not so big that the empty space is intimidating. It's amazing how easily people draw in spite of their initial hesitation and lack of confidence. It is as natural to draw as it is to move. A professional, skilled ability as a visual artist is not necessary in this work. In fact, it can sometimes be a barrier to a more spontaneous and real expression.

Sometimes, while activating this process, an image may come first and then the embodiment will follow. For example, a young man made a drawing of a powerful warrior. When he tried to dance the warrior, his legs were like spaghetti. He just couldn't find a powerful movement in his legs. With his partner coaching him, urging him on, repeating back to him the words he wrote: "I fear thee not," he finally found the power behind his movement, and a conviction in his voice. Through the image he discovered a part of himself he had never experienced before, which gave him enormous strength in facing his fears.

D A N C E

We have looked at movement, feelings and emotions, and imagery under three separate headings. This is misleading because actually the three levels of awareness just described cannot be separated. They function together, though we can focus on one aspect over another when we are teaching. This artificial separation helps us cultivate a larger range in each level of awareness. Ultimately, however, these aspects are integrated. When the three levels of awareness unite in our bodies and through movement, we will make dances with the power to heal. These dances will be special because they are uniquely our own. They come from our direct movements, feelings/emotions, and images, and because of this, they are unique and representative of our lives.

This integration of the three levels of awareness is a process that generates creativity, through the act of dancing. Dance and the creative act are stunning in their application to healing for many reasons:

- Cancer cells are manufactured in our bodies; they are not a foreign invasion from the outside. Just as there are no two people in the world exactly alike, no two bodies are exactly alike. Because of this, cancer cells are also unique to our bodies. This makes cancer difficult to treat: there is no one treatment which works for everyone. Treatment needs to be targeted to the specific needs of the individual. This is a powerful indication that the dance experience needs to be approached as a creative process enabling each participant to express herself, rather than following a pre-conceived formula or pattern imposed from the outside. When we do our dances and they come from ourselves, they are unique and will adapt to our needs. We can create dances that work for us because they come from our bodies and our particular illness. Dance that is approached creatively allows for and encourages this perfect adaptability.

- Dance as a creative act reaches an important state of objectivity. Over and over, I hear the pain and suffering that participants arrive with when they come to class. When they leave, there has been a great transformation. Something has changed. Through an experience of our creativity, we have the opportunity to break the chain of identifying ourselves with our suffering. We are often released from our identification with our suffering by the creative act of a dance which reveals, externalizes, and clarifies our experience for others to witness. This does not imply denial; it implies a new perspective. I like to think of the act of creation as giving birth to a myth—a primary, life-giving act. Since in creation myths we are all created in the image of God, the great spirit, Allah, Buddha, Shiva, the stars, the earth, the life force—whatever that great mystery is that connects us all to each other, all living creatures and the earth herself—when we dance, we are the mystery and the creative principle.

- Dance engages our whole being. It is, in my opinion, the most powerful of the arts because it is holistic in its very nature. Our body is our instrument. It is immediate and accessible, holding our wisdom and truth. We use all of our senses when we dance. We move, make sounds, sing, chant, draw, write. Perhaps this is why the anthropologist Kurt Sachs said, "Dance is the mother of the arts." In dance, all the arts are engaged. By experiencing this integration through dance, we can also experience the artist as a whole, integrated person. We are all artists by nature and do not need years of specialized training to be dance-artists. We all move, respond, feel, and create. This is the basic belief in this approach to expressive movement: it is inclusive. Everyone can do it.

SUMMARY

God guard me from the thoughts men think

In the mind alone.

He that sings a lasting song

Thinks in a marrow bone.

— WILLIAM BUTLER YEATS

This approach to teaching movement is based on the belief that when we begin to use the language of movement rather than the language of words, a different kind of image and emotion arises, which bypasses the controlling and censoring mind. Words label what we already know; expressive movement reveals the unknown. Sensations, feelings, emotions, and images that have been long buried in our bodies are revealed through movement. This is also useful for shifting old patterns, habits, and destructive belief systems. In this book, I will describe some of the methods and activities that help participants enter into a dance that can lead them to a personal transformation.

At the time of this writing, it is ten years since I walked into the Cancer Support and Education Center to explore the ways dance and healing are connected. I have learned much from listening to those who have participated; by responding to their fears and terror through dance; by witnessing their anguish and tears through dance; by supporting their confusion and anxiety through dance; by experiencing their grief and loss through dance; and by rejoicing in their courage and victories through dance. I have learned much about the power of groups where everyone coaches and urges a member who falters or is depressed, where each person shares their story and by doing so, adds to each of our stories. There is power in community when people take great risks to show themselves and their illness, and the community responds with loving support. I have done my own dances when I felt saddened by the death of another person in my life, or the excruciating joy of one more person's triumphant survival. Through it all, I have always remembered to return to dance as an affirmation of my will to live. I believe this is the strongest lesson I have to impart to people who participate in this work: dance and renew your life force.

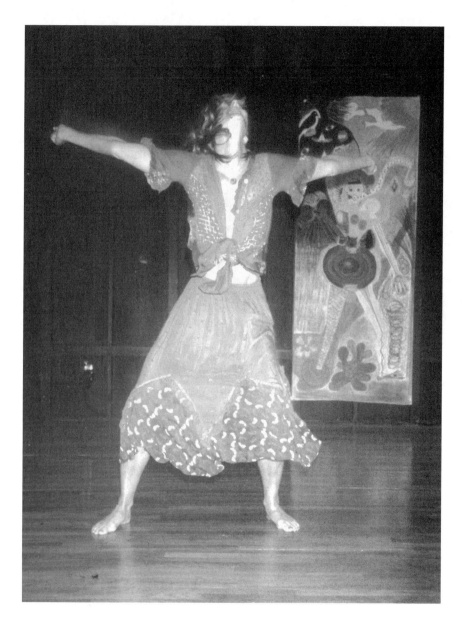

Affirming a will to live.

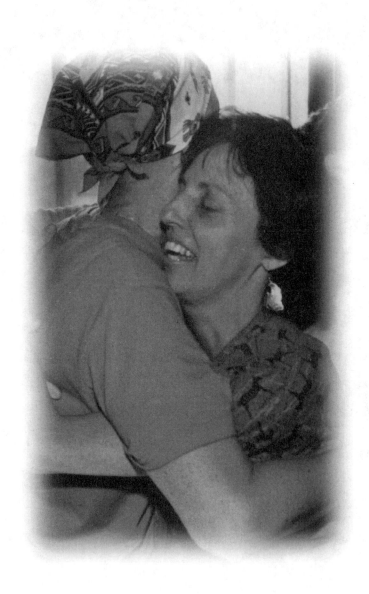

This book is organized into sections, which introduces each of nine lesson plans based on a different theme. Each theme touches upon a life issue that is of special concern for people living with cancer. Each theme will generate a different quality of movement and emotional response. The lesson plans are based on my personal experience in teaching this material and were chosen because they represent pertinent themes. I must emphasize that they are to be used as guidelines rather then hard and fast rules. Themes will change as your class progresses and new themes will arise from the needs of the group. No class could possibly be repeated in exactly the same way because no two groups are the same. Often, I set out with a carefully prepared plan and after class I am surprised at the way this plan has altered. One must go into teaching with this assumption: that what is planned will shift to meet the needs of the moment.

Use the material in this book to generate your own creativity as well as that of the group. You will need to DO the activities yourself before you attempt to teach them to others. This will help you understand the full potential of the work, how it affects your body, your feelings, your emotions, and your images, and how all of this relates to issues in your life. Your personal experience is essential. How else will you know if it is a true path for you to walk with others? You will find greater motivation if you can find a friend to work with. This will give you a context in which to discuss and explore more deeply these lesson plans and their effects.

Your own enthusiasm and belief in the power of dance to heal is a strong factor in how effective this work will be with your students. The late Brendan O'Regan conducted a fascinating research study that illustrates this point. During one of his lectures, he spoke of a chemotherapeutic agent called cisplatinum which was greeted with great enthusiasm. Doctors were getting 75% effectiveness when administering it to their patients. Over time, doctors further removed from their initial enthusiasm for the drug would administer it in a more routine sort of way, and the effectiveness rate dropped to about 25%. This story is relevant to those of us guiding others—we must be truly enthusiastic about our work and project this enthusiasm to our students. This is why you need to *experience* the truth that lies in this kind of movement practice—then you will be genuinely convincing. I used to believe that unless I knew why something worked I could not teach it. Now I believe I don't have to know all the facts, but I do have to know the truth that lies in personal experience itself.

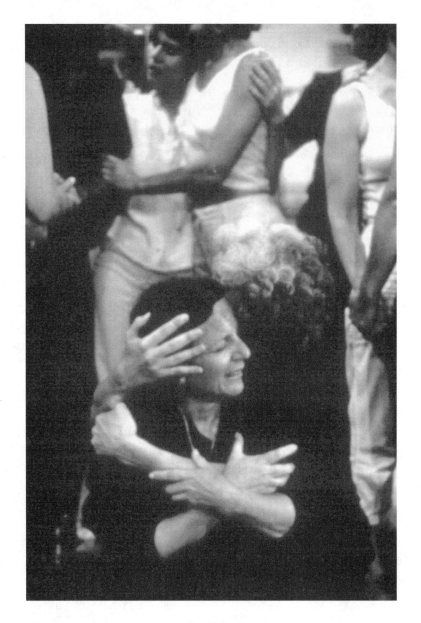

If I can stop one heart from breaking.

The focus of this book is on intimate group classes that are individually oriented. At the end of the book there is a brief description of how to use dance in a community setting. Community healing is very powerful and I believe we need to engage much more attention to this area as well.

Throughout the book the pronoun "she" is used rather then "he" or the more complex "he/she" or "s/he." Each lesson plan is designed for a three-hour session. If you have less time to conduct your sessions, I suggest that you use less of the material rather the cutting short the time for each exercise. Although this material is presented for a group context, it can also be applied in a one-on-one situation with adults and children.

T E A C H E R O R S T U D E N T ?

If I can stop one heart from breaking

If I can ease one life the aching

I shall not live my life in vain

— E M I L Y D I C K I N S O N

Teachers, and therapists of all kinds, we need you. People in the art world: dancers, musicians, painters, sculptors, actors, poets, writers, performance artists, we need you. We need you to turn your practices of art and the imagination into tools for healing. And I believe you need us. Those who have lived through the trauma of facing death gain insight into life. The courage, dignity, and commitment of people who have cancer and other life-threatening illnesses is an inspiration, and a lesson to all of us. You may well find yourself as much the student as the teacher.

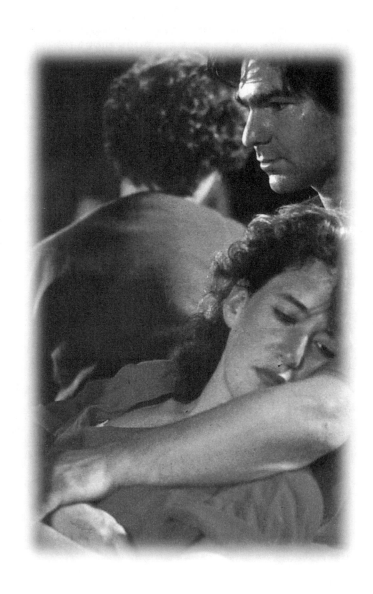

The configuration of a typical class might be an average of fourteen men and women. The make-up of the group consists primarily of people living with cancer. Participants are encouraged to include their loved ones, their friends, or their care-givers. A doctor and several nurses might also be attending. The age range can be from early 20s to 70 years old. The members usually have had no previous dance experience. They come to the class because of a newspaper story, a flyer, a mailing, or a recommendation from a cancer center, conference, or friend. Usually there will be many more women than men. Dance has been relegated largely to the realm of the "feminine" in white Western culture. As a result, heterosexual men often consider dance to be an art form inappropriate for them. Yet, the men who do participate not only enjoy the sessions but find them as useful as the women do.

Venues for these classes may include:

- An outdoor environment in the natural world

- An indoor environment with a clean, warm, spacious floor

- A small living room space with chairs

- A large room in a hospital

Each of these environments can be both a limitation and an opportunity. Certain exercises cannot be done in some spaces; this limitation requires new inventions and creativity on your part. For example, you may not be able to use the floor space in one venue, but chairs will be available. I designed a series of movements in response to this type of situation, which provided many new resources. I found them so useful that now I use them even when it isn't necessary. When first I was informed that this series was to take place in a hospital setting, I was appalled. I thought of hospitals as cold and indifferent places, but after meeting there for a few sessions, and changing the space with the energy of our experiences, the hospital felt like a warm and friendly place. Find a way to work comfortably in whatever space is available to you.

TOOLS

The materials you will need for teaching are as follows:

1. Newspaper print pads, 18" x 22." It is a good idea for each person to have her own pad and to keep track of her drawings from week to week.

2. Materials for musical accompaniment. Instruments like rattles, drums, bells, tambourines, and wood-blocks are nice to have if you work in the same place each week. You will need an audio system for CDs and cassettes.

3. I recommend that each person bring her own journal for writing.

4. Suggest that participants wear loose, comfortable clothes.

BEFORE THE CLASS BEGINS

There are a number of things you will have to do to start your class.

1. Make an attractive flyer describing the class. If you can, have a personal conversation with each participant before the class begins. This will give you an opportunity to be in mutual alignment around expectations.

2. Have participants bring a pad, sheet, or blanket to lie on.

3. The economics of the sessions are an important issue and decisions in this realm depend upon what you want to achieve and who you want to attract. You can solicit outside funding in the form of a grant or a philanthropic donation that will cover the major costs of the program. You can then offer classes on a sliding-scale basis because you are not dependent on tuition to cover costs. Or you can cover costs through tuition and charge a professional fee. The third option is to volunteer your time and use a community space that will not require rent.

4. Be clear with your directions to the place, and the time when class will begin. Honor people's time by starting when you announced you would and stopping on time unless your group agrees to stay longer.

It is part of your job as the teacher to make certain that the room is prepared, neat, clean, and in every way attractive, and that the materials to be used are in order before the participants arrive. Make sure the air is fresh and the room temperature is right. You will need privacy, and soft lighting. The quality of the setting will create a mood for the class. As you prepare the room, place the stools, chairs, or pillows in a circle. Arrange flowers or special decorations before the participants arrive, and if you wish, play music to set the mood you want to convey. Reflect a care for the space, and the comfort and aesthetic sensibilities of the participants. The room where you dance should be a nurturing place. This preparation can help establish a ritualistic or ceremonial feeling among the participants.

It is important to establish trust in the group. Once your class is under way, the participants begin to reveal themselves through their dances, drawings, and stories and will build trust and intimacy with one another. If there is some reason to have a visitor or new person enter class once you have met for a few sessions, speak to the class beforehand to make certain that this is agreeable to everyone. People start to expect a certain situation in class, and are often disrupted by significant changes, such as the addition of a new student, or the absence of another. When people are absent from class, call them to find out how they are, and report this back to the others. It is crucial that the safety of the members of the group is honored. This allows participants a greater freedom in their expression of intimate and often painful material. Sometimes at the end of a class series, after people have gained confidence in themselves and the process, you may want to involve a group in a simple demonstration or an open class. This is one way to share the work they have done with their families and friends. It can be a real boost to the participants and will generate self-appreciation. This is, as well, an excellent way to introduce the work to new people, but it must be something the participants want and agree to do.

THE NEED FOR ASSISTANTS

This is one class situation in which an assistant is very helpful. In a class of this nature, where the experiences of participants are often painful and their needs are demanding, it is important to have extra support. An assistant can be someone who either knows the work very well, has skills in expressive arts and movement, and/or therapeutic skills. It can be someone who has taken the class and is doing it again.

An extra hand is so important. Here is an example of why: one day everyone in the group seemed to be in a similar mood except one woman. As she described her constant and agonizing pain to us, she completely broke down and began to sob. At that moment, it was helpful to have an assistant who was able to take her aside, hold her, comfort her, and focus on movements of relaxation on a one-to-one basis. This was not what the group needed, but it was exactly what this woman needed. When we are able to attend to the needs of all the group members, each person in the group feels supported. By the end of class, this woman was able to rejoin the group. She told us that she had just needed to be held and allowed to cry, and that after the relaxation exercises, she felt much better. The whole group acknowledged her, and felt good that she had been given special attention. They received what they needed, and so did she.

Sometimes an assistant will do hands-on work for those in the group who need one-on-one attention. An assistant can help with the mechanical and logistical details of the class so that the teacher can keep her concentration on the flow of the session without interruptions. There is an incredible concentration required of a teacher in this situation. You must be aware of the participants' response to the material being presented, and be able to react effectively by making changes or adding new ideas. Sometimes a teacher may miss something that an assistant will pick up. Consider yourself in a collaborative relationship with your assistant.

CREATING RITUAL SPACE

The role of ritual and ceremony can be an enriching dimension in this work. Think of ritual and ceremony as something available to you in everything you do. You do not need to borrow and imitate traditional rituals from other cultures or look for something esoteric. Notice the potential ritual in your everyday experience; it can be found in the most ordinary events. I call this "ritual consciousness"—it is a way of shifting awareness from an automatic, habitual way of living your life to one of active awareness and to using dance with the purpose to heal. Ritual and ceremony can happen anywhere at

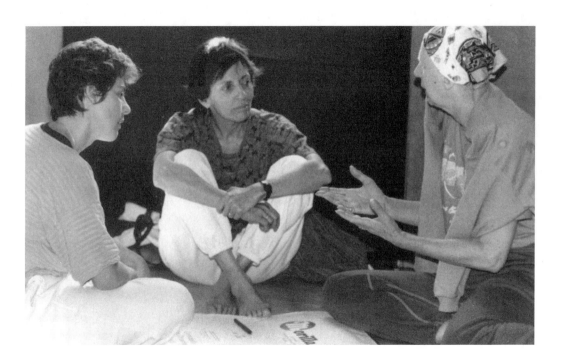

Listen not only to the words but to the tone behind

the words, and observe the body language.

any time. Creating dances that change and transform our lives can be called rituals in the way I am using this word. You will read of many ritual dances in the following pages of this book.

A way to create ritual is to invest the objects of our daily lives with new significance. Let me give you an example. Stones are wonderful objects. On the last day of a class series when the group will part and disperse, you can ask them to bring to class a stone that fits into the palm of their hand. Then, during your closure, pass the stones around the circle so that each person in the group holds each of the stones and says a personal prayer for the person to whom it belongs. When they take their stone home, they will have the remembrance of everyone's prayers. In another scenario, someone in the group is about to go into the hospital. The group could focus on a stone or any object which each person in the group could invest with a personal prayer and she could take that stone with her to the hospital for strength and good luck. Another stone ceremony: throw a group of stones onto the ground, then "read" the symbolic significance of her arrangement. Everyone's interpretation of the symbols of the stones will refer to her own personal story, her own unique perspective.

SPECIFIC ELEMENTS OF EACH CLASS

There are some specific activities you can do in each class, and in a specific order.

The check-in circle at the beginning of each session is a time to listen to each other. Dr. Rachel Remen, in her beautiful book, *Kitchen Table Wisdom*, tells us a story called "Just Listen." In it she says, "I have learned to respond to someone crying by just listening. In the old days I used to reach for the tissues, until I realized that passing a person a tissue may be just another way to shut them down, to take them out of their experience of sadness and grief. Now I just listen. When they have cried all they need to cry, they find me there with them." Later in the story she says, "A loving silence often has far more power to heal and connect than the most well intentioned words."

Here are some ways to listen and empathize:

- Listen not only to the words but to the tone of voice behind the words.

- Observe the body language.

- Avoid giving advice.

- Avoid making any judgments, just accept what the person is saying.

- Give the other person your full attention.

- Avoid interrupting and telling your own story. This is a distraction.

- Reinforce listening by feeding back what you hear and witness.

Carl Rogers, the father of active listening and the patient-client theory, has written extensively on this approach.

There are more ways to listen, which you will discover as you begin to practice. Remember, having cancer will change the way you relate to other people. Very often you do not want to be a burden to your friends and family so you hide behind false smiles and a brave stance. But being with others in a sharing circle who are in the same situation allows you to speak without having to explain or even protect others from your suffering. It is a very special time and as the teacher, you need to provide an open environment where people can do this kind of listening and sharing with one another. Allow each person (or participant) to tell her stories. It also helps to remember that expressing yourself in movement, drawing, poetry, stories, dreams, or insights often says more than ordinary words do. When a group anticipates this time each week, they begin to look forward to it and come with special ways to share. Participants will open up their stories to one another and a bond will begin, which will deepen as they continue to meet. This bond develops into trust and intimacy, which enables all of them to become more creative and open about their emotional needs throughout the series.

Checking-in also provides the leader with clues about how to help people individually, as well as how to present the material for the session or adapt new material to fit the needs of the group. Once I planned to work on up-beat movements requiring a level of physical stamina. After the check-in, I realized this was not appropriate for the group because each person had mentioned that she felt tired and drained. I altered my plans for the day and we worked on relaxation instead until their energy shifted and they were ready to engage in more active movements.

After checking-in, do a sensory awareness activity that moves people from the realm of listening (outside) to the realm of sensation (inside). Cultivating sensory awareness is the first step toward inhabiting the body, and the first step toward bringing participants into a new appreciation of their movement, their bodies, and their dances. Two fundamental sensations are the breath and the pulse. The responses to these two basic principles in movement are endless, as you will learn as you read the lesson plans.

Movement resources follow sensory awareness. The movements you explore should be the resources for the theme of the session and provide material for the participants to use in developing their dances. For example, if the theme is the confrontation of our demons, find ways to lead people into assertive, aggressive, strong, and powerful movements. If the theme is prayer, structure movements around that theme. You need to be able to provide a basic range of resources without dictating a formal way that the movement is patterned or used. Although the movements must not dictate formal use, they need to be precise enough to generate the feelings and emotions appropriate for the theme. For example, intense pounding movements are not going to generate soothing, gentle feelings any more then soft flowing sustained movements will generate anger or determination. This is important to remember when you are structuring your classes. We are looking for expression and congruency in our emotions and our movements.

Each session leads to the culminating moment when each participant creates her own dance. A theme has been selected and explored previously, and by this point in the session, participants have entered their bodies through sensory awareness and collected movement resources around that theme. Now they have the opportunity to express their individual, personal responses by creating their own dances. A dance can range from one to ten minutes, and can include poetry, narration, and music. Participants write stories or poems and make drawings either before or after they dance, according to the realizations and insights of their dances. Associations between the dances created and their connection to our healing process and our lives are shared in a discussion following our dances. We take what we have danced into our lives, and the following week

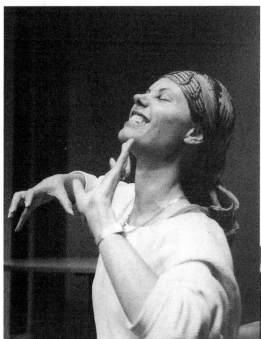

The joy of spontaneous expression.

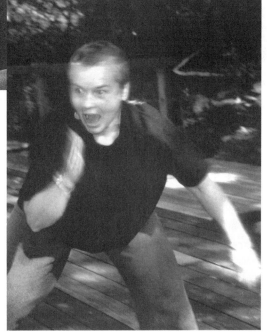

Humor and fun are healing.

we often report on how we were able to use the material of the class in our daily lives. A check-out at the end of each session allows each person to tell if they are ready to leave, or if something has come up during the class that they need to process. Sometimes it may be sadness and grief, but just as often, feelings of empowerment and satisfaction are shared. Sometimes the leader may feel that a person is stuck and needs help in going deeper with feelings. More time can be focused on that person, with the leader feeding back feelings and content in a manner that will help the person take these issues to a deeper level of resolution. This can be done in movement rather than words.

During the check-out, if there is someone or several people in the group who are having a particularly difficult time, invite them to stand in the center of the circle to receive our love, care, and blessings. Here is a way to approach this: Everyone in the circle surrounds the person sitting or standing in the center. Breathe the breath of life into your cupped hands, turn the palms toward the person in the center, and imagine healing light or color radiating from your hands streaming toward and bathing the person in the center. See the person in your mind's eye as vital and healthy. One or two people from the circle can move slowly toward her and softly place their hands on her body. More people can join. You can add a humming sound, words, or light stroking. Receive the person back into the circle. Then all together, lift your palms over your head. Cup your hands together at the top of your head, and then slowly bring your hands in this position in front of your body. Breathe in and release a sound as your hands fly upwards in the air.

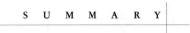

SUMMARY

Each class session includes the following components:

Check-In- Become aware of the overall mood of the participants and the group

*Sensory Awareness-*Enter the body

Movement Resources- Introduce a movement quality and exploration

Take a Break- Give participants a chance to integrate the material before presenting something new

Create a Dance- Discover your own personal expression of the material

Write, Draw, Share- Find connections to your life

Come to completion

The following chapters will give you more specific information about how to apply this method of creative movement to working with people with cancer. I have selected themes I experience as essential, but mine is not, by any means, a definitive list. I have organized the material so that you can see the full structure of each session. Again, I want to encourage you to use this as an inspiration for your own work. Remember to remain creative in your teaching and aware of the people in your classes. They will tell you what they need and where to go.

TAKING CARE OF YOURSELF

I would like to suggest a way to use this book. I suspect that most readers are people in the helping professions. I imagine you experience burnout from always being on the giving side. Now you can switch roles for a change and be a helper to yourself. My suggestion is that you read one chapter of this book at a time, or even one exercise at a time, and then do it. Experience what it brings up for you, reflect upon it, and take this in as nourishment for yourself. You can always come back to the material and study it for its practical applications. Do that later. And start this moment. Don't even try to read the next chapter until another day.

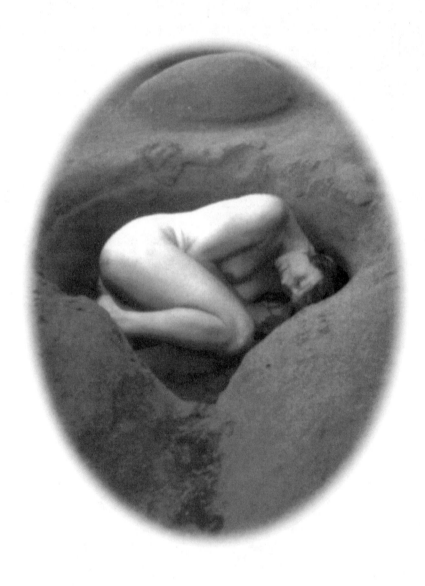

"A person's ability to move is probably more important to his self-image than anything else."

— M O S H E   F E L D E N K R A I S   *from* **Awareness Through Movement**

Many people who are seriously ill view their bodies with shame and distrust and harbor a feeling of being betrayed by their bodies. They often want to escape from these feelings, and begin to depend completely on outside help as a way of escaping their pain. I know from my own personal experience with cancer that the body has an amazing amount of intuitive knowledge and insight that no one else can experience for us, so this dependency on others only weakens our will to live, and our capacity to survive. Our bodies have evolved throughout the ages and represent millions of years of growth and accumulated wisdom. Imagine this potential. This is our inheritance. Everything that we are and could become is housed in our bodies. The mind, the heart, the soul, and the spirit is the body, not separate from it. The power of the integrated body to heal is endless, but we must return to our bodies in order to experience all of this valuable wisdom. No amount of running away will serve us.

The intention of the first meeting is to help participants begin to inhabit their bodies, and begin the journey into the body's endless mysteries. To provide a creative environment to do this, we need to find ways to help participants feel comfortable, safe, and confident. The leader and assistants need to create a rapport with the group in this first session, and the group members need to gain some familiarity with one another. This is the day when all of our relationships to one another, the environment, and the work itself, will begin, so it is necessary to plan carefully this first class. Remember to speak to all the members of the group before this first meeting. This will help you gather details about their specific situations.

C H E C K - I N

In the first class, ask each person to speak about the nature of her illness and what she hopes to gain by coming to these sessions. The session begins with everyone sitting in a circle, and sharing as much or as little as they wish. Telling our stories and revealing our feelings without worrying about being a burden to our families and friends is a great comfort; caring for one another begins here. The teacher models this process by not only sharing her intention in teaching the class, but also her feelings in the moment, or something about her own history that relates to healing. Be brief, honest, and open. Get right to the point and establish guidelines to avoid long periods of talking.

As the series progresses, it is possible to come up with variations on the check-in structure. For example, you can have the group check-in with a partner, and then have the partner report back to the whole group. Or you can have people check-in with simple sentences, gestures, or images that reflect their experiences in the moment. Be alert to the atmosphere in the room and people's behavior, and let these clues help you structure the check-ins and the rest of the class. The purpose in this session is to introduce the expressive and creative qualities of movement, and to begin a self-discovery process beyond the traditional "imitate the teacher" mode. The movement exercises will establish these guidelines as ways of perceiving and experiencing movement.

S E N S O R Y   A W A R E N E S S

1. Find a place in the room where you can stand. Feet are parallel, shoulder-width apart. Close your eyes. Keeping your eyes closed will intensify your awareness of your internal sensations.

2. As you stand, notice how your body is aligned. Sense a straight line dropping through the center of your head, traveling down through the center of your spine, through your perineum, arching over to your hip joints, continuing through your thighs and the center of your knees to your ankles, through the center of your feet, and into the ground. Stack your head, shoulders, ribs, hips, legs around this center line of gravity and sense your balance around this line.

3. *H e a d :* Begin to imagine that your body is dissolving. Start with the crown of your head slowly falling forward, let your eyes drop into your eye sockets. Let go of the flesh of your checks, and let your lips drop forward away from your teeth. Allow your tongue and jaw to release and imagine that you are breathing out through through the back of your head at the base of your skull. At the same time, let your chest collapse.

4. *Shoulders:* Continue dissolving. Let your shoulders fall forwardand give in to gravity while keeping close to your center line. Sense your shoulder blades opening in your upper back as you fall forward. Let your head lead. Follow the pull and weight of your shoulders, arms, and head. Your arms, are now hanging in front of you. Your head, upper arms, lower arms, and hands hang heavy. On each exhalation, release through your spine.

5. *Middle Back:* Continue to fall forward and down, staying close to your center line. Notice that your hip joints will begin to flex. Keep your palms at the same level as your knees, and depress your lower ribcage into your back. Breathe and release through all the vertebrae in your middle back.

6. *Lower Back*: Continue falling down, and begin to bend your knees until they are at about the same level as your elbows. Breathe into your lower back. Your hands will touch the ground. Breathe and release. Become aware of the sensations of your body.

7. Very slowly, reverse this movement and rise up. Press down through your legs and feet into the earth, breathe in deeply, passing gradually up through your lower back. Take another breath into your middle back, then your upper back, and finally into the crown of your head. Feel yourself rise up and lighten.

8. Repeat the exact same movement, only this time focus on the sensations along the front of your body rather then your spine and back.

9. Repeat a third time and focus on the sides of your body rather than its front.

10. On the fourth time, focus on your whole body, sensing the interconnections.

11. The last time, go down faster and dissolve into the ground. End lying down on the floor on your back.

12. Let out a great sigh and relax.

For those who find the standing position too strenuous, the above exercise can be done sitting in a chair. Another option is to present only the first falling and rising section and to do the other parts during another lesson. The most important aspect of this exercise is to help the participant, focus their attention on the sensations in their body as they move. Be specific. Focus on each vertebra, sensing the feeling of expansion and release through the breath.

B R E A T H   A W A R E N E S S

All the movements we do throughout this series are derived from one of the fundamental movements of life: the breath or the pulse. We start with an awareness of the breath. The purpose of a breath meditation is to shift the focus from your external environment to the landscape of your inner body, and to enter into an awareness of your physical sensations and feelings. Using the breath as a pathway can be a form of meditation. Clearing the mind from extraneous thoughts and entering into a pure state of awareness alters brain wave patterns, which induces a state of receptivity and calm.

The essential nature of the breath occurs in four intervals: an inhalation; a pause at the top of the inhalation; an exhalation; a pause and an emptiness at the bottom of the breath. Linger in this emptiness and wait for the breath to return of its own accord. Imagine your breath as an ocean wave. The rising of the wave is the inhalation, followed by a peak and a pause before the wave drops and flows out into the sea. The breath is part of the automatic system, it has its own life, like the waves being pulled by the tides, lifted and dropped into and out of the ocean.

1. Imagine you are lying on warm sand, which molds to fit the shape of your body and gently supports you. Rest in that image.

2. Rub your hands together to warm your palms. Place your cupped palms over your eyes to keep the warmth in and the stimulation of the light out.

3. Breathe in through your nostrils and out through your mouth. Repeat this several times until you do not have to think about it. Relax and move slowly.

4. Begin to massage your face by following the contours of the bones in your face.Experiment with different degrees of pressure from light to hard. Explore your face and your ears with your hands, removing tension wherever you find it. Move your hands on your scalp and loosen the skin.

5. Use your hands like a fine sculpting tool to mold your face. Imagine your face is soft clay and your hands are like a fine sculpting tool that can shape and reshape your face in many different ways. Pinch, press, and stroke.

6. Let your hands massage the back of your neck. Keep your head passive and relaxed and use your hands to rock your head from side to side.

7. Rest. Imagine your hands are butterfly wings softly brushing over the skin on your face and neck. Pause, breathe out, and relax.

8. Remove your hands from your face and notice how your face and head feel. Imagine the pleasurable sensations you feel in your face washing over your entire body.

9. Let the palms of your hands rest on the top of your chest above your breasts and feel the movement of your breath beneath your hands. As you inhale, your chest will rise and expand and fill your hands. As you exhale, your chest will fall and sink and the weight of your hands will drop along with it.

10. Begin to tap along the top of your chest to the rhythm of the beat of your heart (short long, short long), and then tap along your sternum. Imagine these taps as a wake-up call for your body. Brush your skin along your upper chest and softly and gently slide your hands over your breasts until they rest on the sides of your ribcage.

11. Breathe in and expand; breathe out and release. Imagine the movement of your lower ribcage like an accordion. Sense how your ribcage opens and presses into your hands as you inhale, and then recedes and softens as you exhale. Your hands will help guide your attention.

12. Linger in this stillness until your breath re-enters in its own rhythm. Observe this with your witnessing mind.

13. Become aware of the rhythm of the four intervals of your breath. Now try to breathe with your whole body. Roll your spine from the base of your pelvis to your ribcage then back again. Feel your breath flow from your pelvis to your ribs and back down again.

14. Drop your hands to your sides with your palms facing up and notice the sensations in your hands. Do you feel heat or a tingling sensation?

15. Place your hands on a specific part of your body that needs attention. Let the sensations from your hands, which hold the breath of your life, enter and flow deep into the center of this part of your body you are touching.

16. Receive this touch with tenderness. Take your time.

After doing this exercise, which can last anywhere from ten to thirty minutes, you can assume that participants are in a state of awareness that will enable them to take the next step, i.e. to begin to move from a subtle awareness of the motion of the breath into larger gestures and movements. Participants will discover ways to move by relating to the movement of the breath, an essential and continuous rhythm in our bodies. Once people begin moving, you may wish to select and play appropriate music to reinforce their improvisational movement explorations. Encourage people to use the music to complement, rather than direct, their movement. Ask them to initiate movement from their breath as it moves into their ribcage and pelvis. If people are not responding to this suggestion, ask them to start "dancing" by moving only their hands. This will offer enough to help them break the ice and begin.

An awareness of breath and movement can provide a profound experience of deep relaxation. Let the exercise go on for as long as necessary. This exercise can provide a respite from worry and responsibilities, while redefining the body as an oasis of pleasure, rather than the site of pain. This may be an utterly new experience for participants, and one that they will need time to integrate. It may be difficult to move on to any other activity because they may want to stay in this place of peacefulness and calm forever. The purpose of the breath exercise is to shift our focus from the external environment to the body within: to enter into a process of attending to physical sensations, using the breath as the pathway. The mind becomes a witness rather then a controller or director. This is a very comforting place to be. Allow the exercise to come to completion and then take a break.

R E C E S S   T I M E —
A   T E N - M I N U T E   B R E A K

Allow students to rest, talk to one another, write, draw, walk outside, or eat a light snack. People need a moment to absorb the previous activities and assimilate this information into their bodies.

T H E   P U L S E

When the group returns, switch to a movement that contrasts with the breath: the pulse. Have fun, energetic music playing as the group returns. This will create a high-energy atmosphere. Without speaking, initiate holding hands and make a circle.

1. Let the leader spontaneously begin to do a pulsing movement and non-verbally ask the group to join.

2. Stand firmly on your feet, relax your body, and initiate a pulsing movement by bouncing from your knees and allowing the impact of this bounce to travel through your whole body.

3. Check that your knees are directly over the feet rather than turning in or out.

4. Spread your toes apart and balance the weight of your body evenly throughout the soles of your feet. Contact the ground firmly.

5. Check the posture of your spine. Most people have a natural "s" shape with a slight curve in the lumbar region and the neck. Find and keep this posture, and feel the bounce move softly through your spine directly from the ground to the top of your head.

6. Keep releasing the tension in your body so that the force of the pulse will spontaneously jiggle your shoulders, the back of your neck, and travel freely through the vertebrae in your spine.

7. Experiment with doing the pulse at different speeds. Double the time, triple it, or slow it down.

8. Ask people to improvise and find their own variations. Pick someone out from the group and use a follow-the-leader form, until someone else in the circle finds a variation and the others pick it up and do it together.

9. Rest.

WALKING — MAKING A CONNECTION BETWEEN HEARTBEAT AND PULSE MOVEMENT

1. Feel the pulse in your wrist or neck. When you find it, break out of the circle and begin to walk at the speed of your own heartbeat. Keep walking until everyone begins to discover a common pulse through non-verbal consensus.

2. Join your walk with another person. Walk this way for a while.

3. Break contact and join with someone else.

4. Repeat this until everyone has walked with everyone else in the group. Did you ever hear this story? When you put organic cells in different petri dishes they will beat to a different rhythm, but as soon as you put them in the same dish, they will soon begin to beat together. This is what happens when we move together.

Here's another example of an exercise that works with the pulse as an energizer.

1. Find your pulse either in your wrist or your neck.

2. Use this tempo to regulate the speed and rhythm of your movements.

3. Using your hands, begin to pat yourself gently from head to toe.

4. Lightly pat a partner on her back, legs, shoulders, top of head, hands, feet, etc...

5. Pause, and become aware of the sensations in your body.

6. Then, without a partner, shift your attention to your own posture.

7. Notice how the weight of your entire body is resting through your feet.

8. Move your weight forward onto the balls of your feet, then backwards onto the heels, then from one side of your foot to the other.

9. Sense the entire weight of your body evenly distributed through your feet, which are firmly grounded in the floor.

10. Notice how your body posture is stacked from head to toe.

11. Find a vertical alignment with each part of your body balanced over another part. Your pelvis balances over your legs, your ribs balance over your pelvis, your shoulders balance over your ribs, and your head balances on top of your spine.

12. Again, sense your pulse in your wrist or neck. Notice its rhythm and speed. Begin a pulsing movement in your entire body that matches the pulse of your heart.

13. Soften your knees and begin to bounce. Relax and let the bouncing in your knees vibrate through all your joints and into the vertebrae of your spine.

14. Soften your neck and let your head reflect this pulse with a small shaking movement.

15. Place your hands in front of you and as you continue this pulse, notice that your hands will shake without any effort on your part. The pulse will move your hands.

16. Allow this same phenomena to occur in different parts of your body. The pulsing bounce will create movement in other parts of your body.

As you vigorously pulse and bounce, other spontaneous movements will occur throughout your body. For example, your shoulders will begin to slide up and down as the range of your bounce grows. Allow this movement to move you, and watch how your mind begins to witness this movement. As the pulse and bounce become effortless, you can begin to improvise with vigor or with smaller, easy-to-do movements. Liberate your energy, and let your responses guide your dance. This is stimulating to do with the accompaniment of strong rhythmic music. The music acts as an energizer, which will add more enjoyment, motivation, and stimulus to keep moving for a longer time. This exercise can be done sitting down in a chair if a participant finds it too strenuous to do standing up.

*Partner holds your drawing up as
you dance your image.*

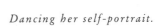

Dancing her self-portrait.

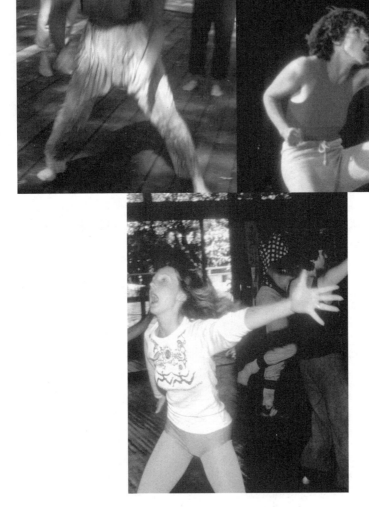

"I am a swirling river."

These can be fun and playful games, as well as opportunities to get to know one another by dancing together. To avoid exhausting participants, be cautious for the first few sessions and go easy with the high energy movement. You can tell by observing the group just how long to do this exercise.

S E L F - P O R T R A I T S

The purpose throughout the series is to bring the members of the group into deeper contact with their personal life experiences through movement and dance, and to separate life-affirming responses from self-destructive ones. The Self-Portrait exercise begins the process of searching for one's personal myths, finding out who we are, which parts of ourselves we can affirm, and which parts we wish to transform for our healing. Give plenty of time for this next process, at least an hour and a half.

P R E P A R A T I O N

We will first do a preliminary exercise to help people overcome their self-consciousness about drawing. So many people will say, "I can't draw," or "I can't dance," or "I can't sing," when, of course, we all can.

1. Take a piece of paper from your pad and select a dark crayon.

2. Hold the crayon in your right hand and lift it in the air. Notice that this movement opens your chest. You will instinctively inhale. Begin to make swirling movements in the air, and without stopping, continue these movements onto the paper. Stop. Look at the lines you have drawn, and see how much movement and life they hold.

3. Turn your paper over and repeat the same thing with the other hand. Try sharp, jagged strokes this time.

4. Take another piece of paper and draw with both hands at the same time.

5. Look at your drawings. Reinforce the lines and add other colors. Play with and intensify this drawing.

You will be surprised at how quickly and spontaneously people will do this exercise. The results are encouraging. We are now ready to begin our self-portrait drawings.

1. Sit or lie down and close your eyes, again returning to your sensations, feelings, and images.

2. In your mind's eye, scan your body from head to toe. Sense your feet, and bring your awareness through your legs to your hips. Sense your whole lower body and then begin to sense your upper body—your back, your torso, your shoulders, arms, neck, and head. Look at yourself from inside and outside. Imagine you are in your favorite place in nature.

3. Pause.

4. When you are ready, open your eyes and make a drawing of your body in your natural surroundings.

5. Write single words that describe what you see in your drawing and group these words into three categories: physical, emotional, and associative. For example, physical words might be: small, swirling, standing, no legs. Emotional words might be: tense, angry, sad. Associative words could be: river, butterfly, or bird.

6. After you have selected your words, give your drawing to a partner. Your partner will hold up your drawing and read aloud the words you have written.

7. Move to these words as your partner reads them to you. Keep referring to your drawing for inspiration for your dance.

8. Switch roles and repeat Steps 6 and 7.

9. Return to your drawing and add any new words that came up for you when you were moving to them.

10. Circle three words that most interest you.

11. Choose one word from each category (physical, emotional, associative). Make a complete sentence out of those three words by adding "I AM..." at the beginning. For example: "I am a swirling, angry river."

12. Partner holds your drawing up for you. Move to these new words, and say them as you move.

13. Repeat your dance over and over. Each time you will go deeper into your dance.

14. Change roles.

By dancing their self-portraits, participants embody physically and emotionally the images in their drawings. They have a chance to actually experience themselves in new and creative ways. The dance will evoke feelings and emotions through the physical dimension. The feelings and emotions that are stimulated are always surprising, exciting, and revealing. Wild demons, loving angels, a sensuous snake, and a flowing river might be some of the images revealed. When we dance these images that well up from our unconscious, feelings and emotions long buried may arise. This is enlivening and there is a healing potential in the discovery of these new and previously unexplored states.

Try this out for yourself before you attempt to lead others in this self-portrait work. Remember to remind participants that there is no right or wrong way to do this process. Your drawings and your dances require no other skill then being present with yourself.

C L O S U R E :   C H E C K - O U T

When all the participants have finished their self-portrait dances, form a circle and give each person time and space to reflect on the message of the self-portrait and what this may have to do with her illness. Ask each person to share with the group her drawing and the sentence she wrote. The self-portrait work is a powerful experience, which will bring up strong emotions. Suggest to participants that they tack their drawing on a wall at home and live with it for a week and let the symbols in the drawing "sink in." Often people will come back the next week with further insights from these drawings.

At the end of the session, stand and hold hands, swing your arms together, and count 1! 2! 3! On 4!, swing your arms high into the air and let out a strong and loud whoop. Take the energy from the whoop and let it cascade down from the top of your head to the base of your pelvis. Different cultures have a different name for this central part of the body—in Japan it is the hara; in Indian philosophy, the second chakra. It is here that we want to gather, contain, settle, and center our energy. If you were to draw a line from your navel through your pelvis to the tip of your tail bone and place a dot in the center of that line, that would be where you can locate this center spot.

S U M M A R Y

In this first class, we begin to make contact with ourselves and one another as a group. Do a leisurely check-in, then an exercise involving the body and the breath, and another with the pulse. This introduces the participants to the basic building blocks of movement. The work with the breath is relaxing; the work with the pulse is energizing. Participants learn to perceive their bodies as a place of comfort and nourishment. Continue with a self-portrait drawing, which each person dances. This dance is an important indicator of self-image and self-identity. End each class with a personal, expressive dance, and a check-out sharing circle.

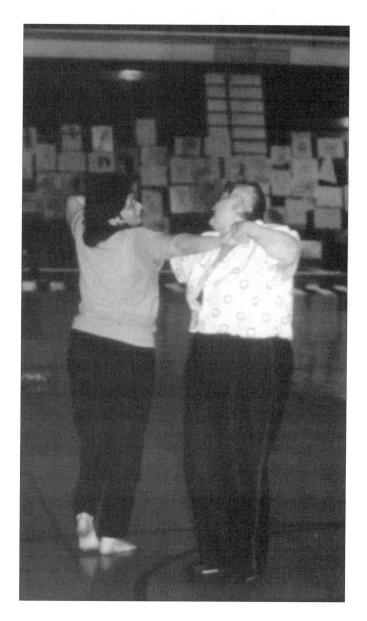

Each class ends with a personal, expressive dance.

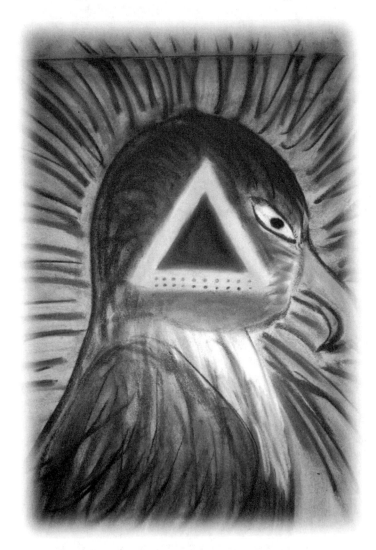

"MY BIRD SYMBOLIZES OPENING UP. WHEN MY BIRD OPENS
HIS WINGS, HIS ANGEL WINGS, I FEEL FREEDOM AND CAN FLY.
I GET TERRIBLE PAINS IN MY NECK AND SHOULDERS
AND WHEN I CALL UP MY BIRD IT STOPS HURTING."

"When a man sought to know how we should live, he went into solitude and cried, until an animal brought wisdom to him. Thus were the sacred songs and ceremonial dances given [to us] through the animals."

— PAWNEE CHIEF, *from Touch the Earth*

This class is based on the notion that people are better able to express their feelings when in the guise of animals rather than as themselves. In this class, we introduce the imagery of animals as potential allies in our healing process. The connection between animals and people found in myths and folk tales stretches back to the beginnings of human existence. The primal bond between animals and humans is so strong that animal dances persist into modern times. From earlier times, we have cave drawings depicting animals as humans, and humans as animals. Something uncanny and perhaps even instinctual happens when we imagine the transformation of our human nature into an animal nature. This action captures the imagination, and inspires us to tap into deep unconscious feelings and psychic needs. When we embody an animal image through movement and dance, we can actually experience and express certain qualities we may not have access to in our ordinary lives.

The socializing force of human society is often repressive, whereas animals express their emotions directly. When a dog is happy, it wags its tail; when excited, it will jump around; when protecting its territory, it will growl; when angry, it will snarl and attack; and when frightened, it will put its tail under its legs and slink away. There is no repression of expression in an animal. By taking on an animal nature, we can come to understand the fierceness of the lion, the strength of the boar, the aggression of the tiger, the playfulness of the monkey, or the patience of the turtle. Embodying the movements of an animal can give us permission to call up censored emotions, or the hidden and blocked emotions that are precisely what we must integrate into our lives as a vital force in our healing.

CHECK-IN

The class begins with a check-in circle with everyone sitting in chairs. The chair is a wonderful prop and you will find that it allows a wide range of movement. Lying down has the disadvantage of the person not being able to see what is going on. Also, it is not always possible to lie down, either because there is not enough room for everybody, or because the floor has not been properly cleaned. And sitting on the floor is difficult for many people, especially men, who have limited flexibility in their hip joints. The position tends to strain the lower back. Standing up is not always possible for people who have physical problems because this position is fatiguing. For these reasons, the chair is perfect.

This session is designed for people of any age, but is especially appropriate for an older group of men and women who have no experience in dance movement, or for people who are physically limited. You might have someone in a wheelchair, or someone who is feeling weak from chemotherapy. Often, a great deal of tension has accumulated around people's shoulders and necks due to stress. Moving the head and shoulders is easier to do in this chair position.

SENSORY AWARENESS IN A CHAIR

Start the sensory awareness exercises by relating to the chair. The chair has a seat, a back, and arms and legs, just as the human body does. It is named after the body itself. Invariably most people are surprised and amused at this connection. Notice how this activity brings the participants into contact with their immediate environment in a comfortable and familiar manner. Ask the participants to sit in their chairs in a way that feels comfortable, relaxed and centered. Ask them to close their eyes and sense their bodies from head to toe as they sit.

Think of this as a game to engage participants in their bodies, their movement, and their feelings. With all of these exercises, give plenty of time between each spoken direction so that people can embody and experience the full impact of each stage of the process.

Watch their bodies and their breathing as clues for your own timing when giving these instructions.

1. Take a deep breath and close your eyes.

2. You and your chair are partners. What do you sense between your body and the body of the chair?

3. Wriggle around in your seat until you find the most centered position between your seat and the seat of the chair.

4. Lean your back against the back of the chair until you sense its support.

5. Place your arms on the arms of the chair, drop your shoulders, and relax.

6. Place your feet directly under your knees so that your lower legs are at right angles to your upper legs. (If someone's legs are too short to touch the floor, get a pillow and place it under her feet.) Your legs are like the legs of your chair. If the legs of the chair are close together, your chair will be pretty unsteady. Place your feet in a way that supports and stabilizes you.

7. Place your knees at the same width as your shoulders.

8. Open your eyes. How do you feel? Are you comfortable? Do you feel supported? Centered? In contact with the chair?

9. Experiment with different ways of sitting in your chair and notice how your posture will affect the way you feel. Tuck your pelvis so that the weight of your body is on your tailbone. Your back will round and your chest will sink. How does this position make you feel?

10. Reverse the position. Lean forward, arch your lower back, and press your chest forward. How does that change your feelings?

11. Cross your legs, and lean to one side. How does that make you feel?

If you notice that the group is involved in this experiment and you have the time, add more resources by asking them to explore positions of their own choosing. Remember to include the feelings which accompany each position. People can also try out each other's ideas, which will take the participants into role playing as well. Experiment with the "bully" when your chest is pushed forward, the "victim" when you slouch, or the "flirt" when you change your arms and legs. Try some explorations of your own and keep a mental record of how your feelings shift as your body position shifts. This exercise will help people understand how physical posture affects emotional state. Many explorations of this kind can be made. A further evolution of the exercise is to respond to your favorite position and become the character that arises in that position.

M O V E M E N T   R E S O U R C E S

1. Close your eyes and take a deep breath. Relax all the muscles around your eyes, forehead, cheeks, mouth. Rub your face with your hands and wipe away all the tension.

2. Breathe out and release the back of your neck. Release your ribcage and your shoulders. Rock from side to side. Your neck muscles will get a good stretch when you hang you head this way. A gentle rocking will ease any strain.

3. Unfold your spine, starting at the base, until your head balances lightly on top of your spine. Breathe in and experience the sensation of lightness.

4. Keeping your head passive, sway your head from side to side, following the momentum of the movement. Let your head be balanced, light, and relaxed.

5. Repeat this movement and let your head drop a little further so that your shoulders drop forward too. Add the sway again.

6. Raise your spine with the inhalation of your breath and notice the sequential unfolding of each vertebra, one on top of the other. Sway again, and this time, leading with your shoulders, twist your body as you sway. Your head is passive, relaxed, and light.

7. Repeat this movement, allowing your head to drop further. Place your hands on your lower back and breathe into your hands. Place your hands on your knees and use them to help you unfold your spine to an upright position. Breathe in.

8. Sway back and forth and let your head be loose like a rag doll.

9. Do the same movements to the right side. Go very slowly. Try to picture what is happening in your spine when you do this. Feel one side of your body flexing as the other side extends. The spaces between your vertebrae open on one side and close on the other. As you come to an upright position, rest and balance your head on top of your spine. Breathe in.

10. Repeat on the left side. Let your head fall to the side as far as is comfortable, letting the weight of your head bend you over. Notice how far along the sides of your body you sense this movement. Notice that your ribcage expands on one side and flexes on the other. Remember to breathe with this movement.

11. Rest.

12. Use the back of your chair for support and tilt your head backwards.

13. Bring your head upright, in place at the top of your spine. Rest.

14. Let your hands brush lightly over your face and rest on your chest. Breathe into your chest and as you breathe in, lift and open your chest. As you breathe out, close and collapse your chest. Include your head in these lifting and dropping movements. Connect to your breath and pause in between.

15. Sense the connection between your head and chest in these movements.

16. Pay attention to the way your shoulders connect to your body. Lift your right shoulder to your right ear. Hold the position, and hold your breath. Release. Breathe out and let go even more. Do you notice any difference between your left shoulder and your right? Look around the circle and see if you can see the difference in your friends. Do the same movement on the other side.

17. Lift both shoulders and then drop them.

18. Reach forward with your shoulders, and then backwards. Do you notice that your shoulder blades slide forward and backwards and that your head will also move forward and back? If your head will not move with your shoulders, try to relax the base of your neck. We are used to holding our heads up with our neck muscles; it takes time to let those muscles relax.

19. Experiment with moving your shoulders around in a circle, one side and then the other. Next, try moving one shoulder forward while the other shoulder moves back. Notice how your spine rotates when you move your shoulders this way. Follow this rotation with your head. Rest.

20. Keep your arms at shoulder height. With your left hand, stroke your body, starting from the center of your chest, and crossing over your right shoulder, upper arm, lower arm, hands, fingers, and out into the air. Follow this movement with your eyes. Keep your seat connected to the seat of the chair and as you move, your spine will spiral. Repeat on the other side.

21. Rest.

22. Move your hands down to your belly and take the movement of your breath into your pelvis. Rock your pelvis forward and backwards. Once you have isolated this pelvic movement, explore different directions in which your pelvis can move. Remain aware of your breath. Move slowly. Make sure that the movement is pivotal, rather than just leaning forwards and backwards. When the rocking movement is pivotal the lower back will arch when you rock forward and flex when you rock backwards. Check this out. This will energize your lower back and free your pelvis.

Another variation of this movement would be to leave the chair and position yourself on your hands and knees. In this position, flex and extend your back and head, and your pelvis will follow. Some people find it easier to do this in the chair, while others work better on their hands and knees. Do this movement side to side, and in a circle. Rest. Then stand up and walk around and notice how your body feels.

PULSE: THE UP-BEAT AND THE DOWN-BEAT

Play drum music with a strong beat to stimulate participants to mobilize their energy. This will help establish a light and jolly mood. The group always enjoys the spirit of dancing together and there is usually lots of laughter and big smiles. It is important to balance serious concentrated movements with joyful and playful ones. One of the most

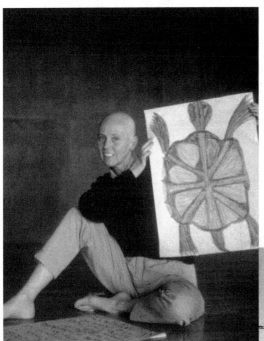

*"My turtle has a hard shell that protects me.
When I was told to get my affairs in order
because I did not have much more time
to live I called upon Great Mother Turtle
to protect me from these crushing words."*

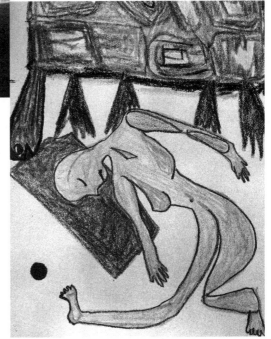

"O Great Mother Turtle, Rescue Me From Death."

effective ways to do this is by exploring our relationship to the down-beat and the up-beat in the pulse. Within this polarity lies a core emotional link to your physical body. People who cannot or will not express anger or power will find themselves experiencing those difficult emotions in spite of their inhibitions when they begin to work with accenting the down-beat. The same holds true with the accent on the up-beat. Feelings of great joy and victory come when this quality of movement is experienced.

1. Remove your shoes so you can feel the earth. Shake your feet one at a time, rotate inwards and outwards, stretch and flex, paw the ground, make a fist with your feet, alternate by opening them out. Stand up and take the beat of the music into your body.

2. Move to the beat in different parts of the body, hands, shoulders, head, and legs. Improvise. Move with another person, or with the whole group. Play with this as long as you can to build endurance.

4. Form a circle, and in the circle, begin to swing your arms. Lift your arms in the air, drop them, and rebound back up into the air.

5. Once this swinging has been established, begin to accent the down-beat of the movement. Let your arms come down very strong on the down-beat. The movement will turn into a pounding or hitting action. Do this solo, and then together. Add a sound on each down-beat. The feelings that match this movement are power, strength, anger, and determination.

6. Now switch the accent to an up-beat and swing your arms up. The feelings that match this movement suggest victory, joy, or happiness.

These are essential emotional movements for the group to experience, especially in preparation for the animal ally dances. Bring this exercise to a completion. After you finish, take a break. When the group returns, pads and crayons should be in place and the chairs moved back to make as much open space as possible for their animal dances.

ANIMAL ALLIES: GUIDED
VISUALIZATION AND DRAWING

This next process is a guided visualization which I use as a way to help people find their animal allies. Prepare the participants by speaking clearly about what will happen next, e.g., "We are going to go on a guided visualization to find our ally who will reveal some message we need to hear. It is a mysterious way of receiving a message but in the mystery lies hidden truths." Find your own way to introduce this material rather than repeating these words. It will be more convincing if you do. Have everyone find a comfortable position and begin to take them on this guided journey. Take enough time to allow people to make the images their own and to find their animals in their own time.

1. Use your breath to enter your body. Breathe deeply and relax.

2. In your mind's eye, imagine a void. Fill this void with a sky, trees, water hole, a vast plain, a mountain, whatever natural environment you imagine. Take your time.

4. Find yourself in this environment. Start looking for a special species of animal. The smells and sounds of the environment are all around you. You are very excited and curious. Discover a place where you can sit down and rest. Although you are resting, you are very alert. Gradually become aware that you are being visited by a creature. Remain still and wait for this creature to come to you. Once it has arrived, begin to make friends with it. Study carefully how it moves, sounds, feels, and acts. Become so engrossed with this animal that you merge with its body and take on its form.

5. You are now this animal. How will you sound? How will you move? What will you do? Find the animal's voice and movement and embody this animal.

6. Interact with the other animals in the environment.

7. When you are finished with this movement exploration, begin to return to your human form.

This part can take as long as an hour or be as brief as twenty minutes. People can become intensely engaged and you can expect a series of things to happen: fighting, playing, cuddling, protecting, etc. Sometimes there will be laughter, growling, or terror.

This exercise can be emotionally charged, but generally people enjoy the childlike and spontaneous atmosphere.

Another development of this exercise is to experience yourself as a human being behaving, responding, and interacting with your animal's characteristics. In other words, you would translate your animal characteristics into human behavior. This can be played out with everyone freely walking through the space, and contacting others in the guise of your "human animal." For example, if your animal ally is a tiger, you could take the energy of the tiger into your interactions with other people, and rather than growling at them or eating them as a tiger might, you would translate this into human behavior and language. This transference can bring your animal image into great immediacy.

DRAWING AND DANCING YOUR ANIMAL

This part of the exercise will take thirty minutes or more.

1. Staying with the mood of your animal, immediately go to your drawing pad and make a drawing of your animal.

2. On another piece of paper, collect movement, feeling, action, and sound words about your animal. What might your animal do, feel, or say?

3. Circle four words you like.

4. Use these four words in a scrambled way to make a chant or tell a story. You can add prepositions.

5. In groups of three, dance your animal allies. One person dances her ally; another assists her by reinforcing or mirroring her movements. The third partner takes the words she has written and narrates or chants them while the other two dance. In all three roles, there is room for improvisation. The words need to be repeated and played with rather than read in an ordinary way.

6. Everybody has a turn and switches roles.

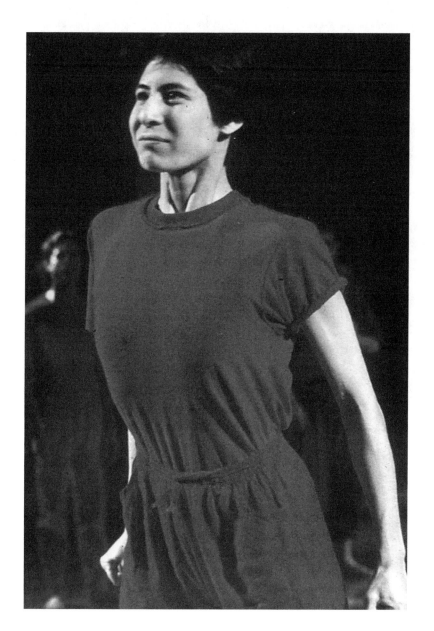

Dignity and well-earned pride; I can handle anything.

7. When you have finished doing this, write down how your animal can be your ally. How can this animal help you when help is needed?

8. Ask your ally a question: How will you be able to help me in dealing with my illness and the other difficult issues of my life? Listen for the answer.

If there are some participants who cannot dance their animals, either out of fatigue or weakness, either invite someone else to do it for them or, better yet, encourage them to find a way to use their hands and face to feel, express, and embody their ally in any way they can, however subtle or invisible it may be. Encourage and coach people. The following are just a few examples of some of the writing and storytelling people did after they danced their animal allies.

Bright spring sunshine makes the California coast look utterly clean and very beautiful. The ocean shifts green blue in restless motion against the rocks and the intimate, small beaches between cliffs. I am swimming with the whales. You might think this would be dangerous for a 59-year-old woman with cancer. But you don't know these whales. There are many of them swimming together, a whole school of whales. I swim among them, feeling their huge bodies around me as we move under the green water. They never bump into me, or hit me with a fin, or slap with me their big tails. They know I'm here among them, a small human body and mind surrounded by their bigness. I feel completely safe among them, protected by their numbers and their bulk. How they sag and wiggle through the water, hump their backs, drive themselves forward with those powerful tails. I try to swim like them. I wiggle and kick my feet. I love these whales and I embrace them. I straddle one small whale and ride for a while. Then I swim between two huge ones, touching their sides companionably. We are going somewhere. My mind says we are going to Baja to give birth to our babies and lie in the sun. But I don't really know where we're going. I float face down, undulating with the wash of water that comes from their movements.

I pretend I am a pregnant whale on my way to Baja. Then I float down to the bottom and stand on the muck. I wave to the whales, pointing out the direction they should go. My arms move around in a circle like a semaphore, directing them. Of course they already know where to go, but they indulge me, letting me wave them forward. Oh swimming, touching, down deep, dark, safe, going on forever, whales, I'm having a whale of a time. I'm going beyond limits, beyond cancer, illness, beyond fatigue and pain, beyond thoughts of tomorrow.

My whales in the ocean are digesting the doctors, technicians, nurses, researchers. They'll all become whale poop soon and float to the bottom of the sea. This is freedom. I let the whales do it all for me. Show me how to swim.

Point the direction to go.

Another animal ally story came from a support person in the group. This young Japanese woman had just come to this country. Soon afterwards, she met and married a man much older than she who has cancer. He is tremendously demanding of her and wants her to take care of him day and night. She is overwhelmed and upset by her situation. In her dance, she visualized a blue bird and when she danced it, she had us all sit in a circle around her. She began doing bird calls. She squawked and requested that we ask her some questions: "What are you trying to say to me, you beautiful blue bird? If you know something I don't know, tell me." Everyone in the group played a role in her dance and asked her these questions. She began to cry softly and finally asked the group for help. She told us she is all by herself, and feels so burdened. In response, members of the group began to make plans to spend time with her outside of class and this began to ease her heartache.

One woman in class was having a difficult time mobilizing her strength to do a particular movement requiring a strong, aggressive stance. We found a way to help her find this movement by first bypassing the emotional association of anger and focusing on the purely physical force behind the movement. As we worked on a swinging movement, she was instructed to add more force to it as she dropped her arms. More and more force was gradually added until her emotions became engaged. She began to pound with her arms and legs. Her whole body became powerful and she shouted, "NO! NO! STOP! OUT OF MY WAY!" She was taking a powerful stance. Later in the session, she drew a giraffe and she danced her story of this giraffe. In her story she wrote that the giraffe was stalked by a tiger who began to run after her. In her dance, she ran around the room as another person danced the tiger chasing her. As she ran, she became panicked and frightened. When we talked about the experience she said, "I was afraid the tiger would kill me but I didn't want to run away. This giraffe is taller and bigger and could confront the tiger and stop him but I don't know how."

She was reminded of the pounding movement we had done earlier and how she had added her voice and shouted STOP on every down-beat. I asked her to do her dance again and when the tiger chased her to turn around and use that pounding movement and her voice. She did the dance again, the tiger chased her, she ran away, and then suddenly she turned around and confronted the tiger with a strong stance and a shout. The tiger, feeling overpowered by her determination and strength, stopped suddenly in her tracks, startled by her unexpected power. Everyone in the class remarked about the change in her posture and expression on her face. She seemed to transform before our eyes from a victim to a self-assured woman. She could apply this new attitude and way of being to confront her cancer. Through movement, she had found a new way of accessing her power.

I must include one last example because it gave so many of us a good laugh. One time when I was beginning a class at the Cancer Center, I was introduced to the group as a movement specialist and dancer. I noticed that a young, attractive woman sitting opposite me responded by quickly crossing her legs in a tight closed position and folding her arms across her chest as she looked down. Before we began the class I asked her what was going on and if she wanted to tell me anything. She said, rather hesitantly, that she hated her body and the thought of moving and dancing terrified her. I listened and we continued on with the class. When it was time to draw our animal ally, I noticed she had drawn a beautiful, well-defined monkey with two bright green balls between its legs. Her dance of this monkey was hilarious as she spread her legs and rocked from side to side as a monkey does. She playfully exposed her "two green balls" and had a great time doing her dance. Her ally reminded her that she was able to have fun and enjoy the sensuality and joy of her body after all. Cancer had not taken that away from her.

SUMMARY

In this session, we find an animal ally to support us in our experience with cancer. Begin with a check-in and a sensory awareness exercise. Start with the group sitting in chairs, and adapt the sensory awareness exercise to this circumstance. Work with strong assertive movements that develop from a rhythmic beat. By accenting the down-beat, participants can experience power and determination. After the group is up and moving, do a guided visualization that leads to our animal allies. Encourage participants to embody this animal, dance it, and then listen to what it has to say. After doing this dance, draw your animals, and write down what you have learned from these allies. This can also be reversed: participants can draw their animals first, write about them, and then dance them using their writings as a narrative score. The class ends with a sharing of the many ways the animal allies can teach us a lesson to apply to our lives.

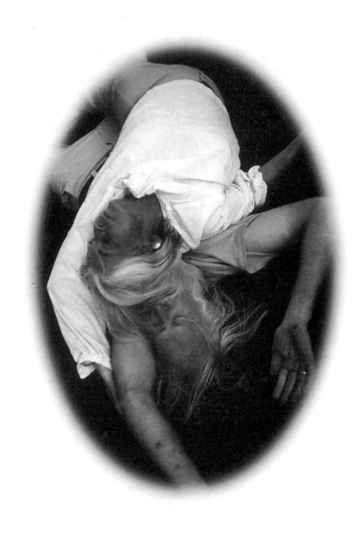

My personal and professional experiences have demonstrated that when
people have sufficient self-awareness to have healthy self-esteem, and when they
promote an open honest climate, much pain can be eliminated. We can eliminate
irrelevant arguments, wasted energy, withholding, lying, undermining, and
other inefficient and misery-producing activity.

— W I L L S C H U T Z *from* **The Human Element**

The quality of our relationships is an important aspect in our lives, and in our healing process. In a time of illness, we need the support of our relationships more than ever. We need to feel connected to others. We need to feel the love and support of our families, and to feel ourselves as part of a group and a community. Some of us need to see ourselves in a larger relationship to the world and to the earth itself. When our relationships are not working, something vital is missing from our lives, something we need to keep our immune systems strong and our spirits high. In a time of illness, we need to be heard without judgment or advice. We need to learn how to stand up for ourselves in a conflict and still respect the other person. We need to learn how to be honest and remain unafraid of hurting other people's feelings. We need to know when to say NO and when to say YES. In short, we need to give ourselves permission to be fully expressive of our true selves. Without this, we create unbearable stress and pain in our lives.

I just received a call from a friend who sounded desperate. She said that her father had cancer and that he wouldn't leave the house, see his friends, or do anything that might lift his spirits. He had essentially given up and was in isolation, depending fully for his care upon his elderly wife and daughter. Perhaps he imagined his friends would not want to be with him. Perhaps he had never had a good relationship and did not realize how much he could receive and what his friends could receive by giving. Many of us have difficulties believing in our relationships, or turning to other people when we are in distress. When we are ill, we must learn to ask for help, and to receive the abundance of love that surrounds us.

The following material can unfold in one class or in a series of classes. Because the issue of relationships is so consequential, I believe you can work on this issue for an entire series. These lesson plans use movement to explore our present relationships and how we might change what is destructive, and reinforce what is nourishing. Often this material helps people see what they have in their relationships, what they need in their relationships, and how to remain true to their own impulses in relating. If you choose to use relationships as only one theme in part of a longer series, use the first lesson plan by itself. The other scores are the evolution of that first lesson plan. It is helpful to infer a metaphoric understanding of movement and dance with this material. In this way, participants can see that the way they dance their relationships in class is related to how they dance their relationships outside of class.

ENTERING THE BODY

This exercise is designed to provide a skill that enables participants to experience the difference between physical tension and relaxation. It is important to know when our muscles are holding on, and when they have let go. This distinction can be subtle, but it is vital for maintaining our health. Even now as I am writing, I took a moment to scan my body and noticed that my shoulders were hiked up to my ears and that I was leaning forward, tense in my back rather than relaxed and using the back of my chair for support. As I dropped my shoulders and leaned back in my chair, my breath came more easily and my feelings shifted. I felt more at ease as I let the tension drop away.

1. Find a comfortable place on the floor. Lie on your back.

2. Inhale and hold your breath for ten counts. Then exhale.

3. Repeat this several times.

4. Place your arms at your sides at shoulder height and lift your right arm one inch from the ground. Hold it there. Count to ten and then let go.

5. Repeat this.

6. Do the same thing with your left arm. When you do, notice how the tension is not only in your arms but in other parts of your body as well.

7. Lift your head one inch off the ground. Hold and count to ten. Then slowly let go. Did you notice the tension reflected in other parts of your body?

8. Repeat this several times.

9. Lift your knee one or two inches off the ground. Hold and count to ten and then let go. Repeat this.

10. Do the same thing to the other side.

11. For more of a challenge, lift both knees at the same time and then let go.

12. For even more intensity, keep your knees extended, and lift your feet off the ground. Then let go. (Don't do this if it is too strenuous on your lower back.)

13. Lift your arms, legs, and head at the same time to experience the maximum amount of intensity, and let go. Melt your whole body into the floor, and relax.

After doing this exercise we have a common vocabulary based on a real experience. We have now sensed what is meant by "tension" and "relaxation." It is an experience, not a concept. You can work on variations of this exercise.

LEVEL I: PASSIVE/ACTIVE (LEADING OR FOLLOWING)

This material is so very rich that I suggest you present it in three parts during three different consecutive sessions. Do this whole series of exercises in partners.

Lying Down

1. One person lies down and closes her eyes. The other person sits beside her.

2. Both take several deep breaths together and establish a rapport with one another.

3. For the partner lying down, let your body become heavy and loose. The sitting partner: lift the arms of your partner, and move them up and down slowly, gradually walking around your partner's body, while still carrying her arms. The passive partner remains loose, heavy, and relaxed. Let your partner move you.

4. Repeat the lifting movement using different extremities of your partner's body, such as the head and legs.

5. After ten minutes or so, switch roles and repeat the same exercise.

Sitting

1. Face your partner.
2. One person will close her eyes (A) and the other will keep her eyes open (B).

3. Partner B begins to lead A. First move A's arms. Then gently place your hands on the side of A's head. Leading from the head, move A in different directions. Finally, hold A by the shoulders and rock her torso. Partner A, relax and allow yourself to be led.

4. Share feelings or images that came up for you. How did it feel to be the receiver? How did it feel to lead?

5. Switch roles.

6. Do the same exercise as before, having switched roles. Based on your own experience of leading or following, you will have more resources to work with. Do you feel different when your partner is leading your arms, your head, or your whole torso? Invent new ways of using your body when leading.

I suggest you do this work very slowly and notice how leading from different parts of the body such as the head, the arms, or the torso will evoke different feeling responses. You may hear a variety of emotional responses to this exercise such as: "I was afraid to let go"; "I wasn't ready to trust"; "I am afraid of being a burden." People also share a variety of images: a mother leading her child, or a child being cared for by her mother. All of these responses invariably resonate with the person's life outside of class.

Someone commented that when she was held by the shoulders she felt more secure than when she was held by the hands. If you observe someone having trouble letting go, you should remember that this may be an emotional reaction but could also be related to her inability to let go. It may be a good time to remind the person of the sensations linked to

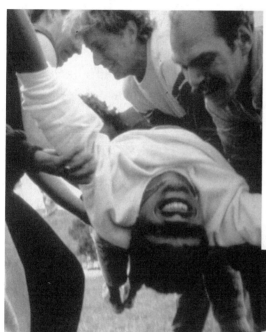

An exercise in trust:
  falling backwards and being caught.
Anxiety turns to laughter.

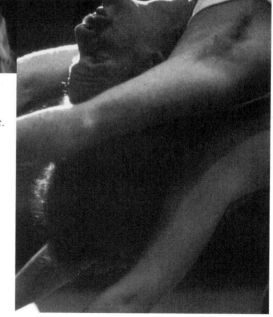

Opening the chest opens the heart.
  Being supported by a partner enables us
to move beyond our usual limitations.

relaxation that were explored earlier in the class. Often a person is emotionally ready to let go but the tension in her body is so habitual that she does not know how. Given time and repetition, the person will soon learn this skill. It is often a revelation to people that you can receive so much support by simply letting go and allowing another person to move you. It is equally surprising to know that the role of leading can be so creative.

There are various ways to share our personal experiences with one another in this exercise. I often suggest that each partner practice listening and then feeding back what they have heard. Here is a good model to follow: "When I experienced _____ movement , _____ feelings were aroused..." Keep listening and feeding back what you hear without advising or judging your partner. Someone might say, "When you led me I felt self-conscious, as if I were a burden to you." Rather than saying, "You shouldn't feel like that. You weren't a burden to me," just listen. Uncomfortable feelings may come up that might tempt you to advise your partner, or try to "fix" things. Remember that there is no problem, and there is nothing to fix. When sharing your own feelings, you might say, "When I was leading you, I felt a deep feeling of warmth and tenderness." This is more important for your partner to hear than any idea you might have about her experiences. Sharing our own truth, no matter what it is, will have integrity and make us feel good about ourselves. Discovering that we were not a burden can be something we need to hear. And this may have analogies in our day-to-day lives—perhaps we have been cutting ourselves off from those around us who want to be supportive.

After sharing together, move on to the next part of the exercise.

Standing in Place

During this part of the exercise, move up and down and side to side, but stay in one place.

1. Partners rise to a standing position. This will engage your legs. Breathe out, and let your breath flow from your upper body to your lower body. Keep your knees soft.

2. Leaders, move your partners up and down, rather than moving into space. Take the liberty to approach your partner from any direction. You may choose to lead from behind, the side, or the front.

3. After you have reversed roles, take time to share your feelings and images. Tell your partner which movements evoked which feelings. Again, practice active listening.

After this, everyone will do a drawing stimulated by this experience, and then share their drawings. Some of the questions you might ask to evoke responses from the participants could be: How did it feel to lead? How did it feel to follow? What images were evoked for you? In the check-out circle, share your drawings as a way to understand how the answers to these questions are applicable to your life. You may be surprised at the connections participants will discover between the movement and their life experiences.

L E V E L I I :
P A S S I V E / A C T I V E

As we continue with scores related to passive and active movement, or leading and following, we are exploring more deeply how we come into relationships with one another, and then how we respond once we are in them. In addition, participants get a sense of their roles in relationship. They can see whether they tend toward activity or passivity, which state they prefer, and which is more challenging for them. They can learn things about how they are, how they would like to be, and what they might wish to change. Some of this learning will refer back to early family issues or primary relationship issues and is often reflected in their relationship to their illness.

Moving Through Space

1. One person works with eyes closed, the other with eyes open. Facing each other, one partner (A) place her hands on top of her partner's hands (B). A is the follower, B is the leader. B walks very slowly, taking care that each step is firmly grounded. When you lead, look where you are going to avoid walking into people, walls, or chairs. Walk forward and backward in a circle. Notice if your partner is breathing easily. A, try to stay light and easy. Give this exercise all the time needed to fully experience moving through space.

2. Change roles. Each partner notice how you feel when you are leading or following. Do you have a preference for one role over another?

After you have done this exercise, reassemble the group in a circle and share how this movement relates to people's relationships. Here is an example of feedback. One woman who had her eyes closed was petrified. She could barely catch her breath. At first she did not have any idea why she was responding this way and then she told us that she was afraid of going blind and becoming dependent on other people. As the story continued, it was revealed that her elderly father is blind. She spends a good deal of time caring for him. She doesn't mind his blindness, but she does resent his attitude and constant dependency on her. Doing this exercise brought up these feelings for her.

Another person stated at the beginning that she did not want to lead. She had nothing but resistance to leading. She didn't want any more responsibilities in her life; she wanted to be led by someone else. I encouraged her to do the entire exercise, and when the roles were switched and it was her time to lead, she was surprised at how much fun it was. Another person loved being led because she said it reminded her of her father teaching her to ballroom dance when she was a child.

After checking-in, do more leading and following. This time the directions can be more complex. Again, work with your eyes closed.

1. Leader: create unexpected situations for your partner. Lead faster or slower; stop and start; experiment more freely with directions and speed.

2. Lead from different parts of the body. Keep experimenting. Take plenty of time.

3. Reverse roles.

This will heighten the intensity in the room. It is likely that this version of the exercise will elicit laughter, gasps, and other sounds of surprise. After you have finished this exercise, make a drawing of what it was like for you. What images or memories or emotions were evoked?

Here are some examples of what people discovered in the movement and the drawing. Virginia has been struggling with cancer in the bridge of her nose and has suffered terrible headaches and eye problems for several years. Her drawing was a large face with closed eyes and an open mouth with the word "AH" coming out of it. She also drew clouds floating across her forehead. After the exercise, she said she felt so released, tranquil, and soft. She loved being led with her eyes closed and had not felt so good in years. Her partner, Janice, drew a picture of two figures. One was a frail young girl with a large red heart for a torso dripping drops of blood. She called this figure "bleeding heart." The second figure had wings. She called this her "guardian angel." Even though she could not have understood how her partner felt about her, Janice could feel on a deep movement level that she was being led by a guardian angel.

LEVEL III: BLENDING

This next section describes a third class pertaining to the theme of relationships as seen through the metaphors of passive and active movement. The next phase is to work with a blend of the two. Blending is a way of moving together without a perceptible leader or follower. It is a rather strange and inexplicable thing, but it does happen that two people can begin to move by focusing on the slightest, smallest movements between them, and begin to simply flow with this movement as if being moved by a force outside themselves. The capacity to move with more complexity will come about naturally as a rapport builds between partners. The results are harmonious and peaceful, even when the partners are using high energy. The most effective way I have discovered to teach this material is to do a non-verbal demonstration with another person. You can do this with one of your assistants, or with one of the participants.

1. Mirror one another's movements without anyone leading.
2. In order to blend with another person, you must stay present all the time. Losing awareness for one instant will cause you to lose contact with your partner.

3. Do this dance until people are tired and ready to stop. At the end, check in with one another about your experience.

The experience of blending with another person can be very exciting. In one class when participants shared their experiences, this was the general feeling. Sandy seemed to be having a good time when suddenly she realized that sadness was coming up for her. She told us that she realized now that the reason she and her partner had broken ties was because her partner was giving her too much pressure during a time when her struggle

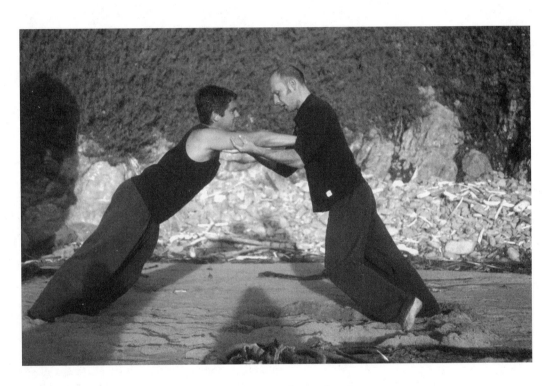

Two people being active at the same time introduces the element
of determination, but also playfulness.

with cancer left her feeling vulnerable. She needed more blending in her life. She had not realized this before and now she felt sad. This is a good example of how someone can understand a relationship in her life outside of class through the metaphors of the movement exercise.

Some other responses to this exercise included: "When we finished, my partner and I were surprised and delighted that we had come up with exactly the same image—we both saw a waterfall. This was a very healing to us both. We do not know how we came up with the same image because we did not talk about it until just now." One participant felt like a child being held by her mother and at the same time like a mother holding her child. Another felt extremely relaxed and energized. She was in a trance-like state where she felt both inside and outside her body at the same time. This was a new and exciting experience for her.

The next week this same woman shared with us a way she applied this exercise in her life. She and her mother have a good deal of tension and conflict in their relationship. One day her mother saw her practicing some movements we do in class and she wanted to know what she was doing. Carol suggested that they move together and she held her hands out for her mother to join her. She played some music and then led her mother in a dance that developed through blending. She told us, with great animation, that this was the most loving experience she had ever had with her mother. I imagined that the movement allowed them to get past the problems of verbal communication and to the core of the warmth and love that exist between them.

LEVEL IV: ACTIVE/ACTIVE

This last relationship exercise will require the entire class time. It is based on two people being active at the same time. A way to present this material is to weave this new element into the others. For example, one person might be leading another who is following, but then the one who is following might shift and be the active leader. Now the two partners would be trying to lead at the same time. This introduces the element of conflict, challenge, determination, and anger, but also playfulness, high energy, humor, and exuberance will appear. This exercise can teach us about the positive sides of assertiveness in relationships.

1. Place your hands against your partner's hands and begin pressing lightly, then increase this pressure until you have reached your limit.

2. Explore using different parts of the body to create pressure: hips to hips, back to back, etc.

3. Now switch to pulling. Again, begin softly and gradually increase the amount of force.

Another activity that could be explored is rhythmic clapping.

1. One person sounds out a rhythm. Partner responds with another rhythm.

2. Play off one another's rhythms.

Any oppositional movement situation can be used to explore the active/active dynamic. This will help people explore tension and dynamics, as they are experienced in relationships, and expressed through creative movement.

1. One person moves in one direction. Partner moves in the opposite direction.

2. Repeat this in different ways. For instance, one person moves up, the other person moves down.

DRAWING YOUR RELATIONSHIPS

At the closure of this series of relationship scores, you can do a drawing of what an ideal relationship might look like. Here are some questions that might stimulate your thoughts before you do the drawing:

• What do you want more of?

• What do you want less of?

- What do you get that you don't want?

- What do you want that you don't get?

As you reflect on these questions, let them influence the way you draw and how you design your dances of these drawings. This can be a satisfying score to dance. Someone could take the part of your primary partner and then the person who designed the score could direct her partner in how to use the elements of passive and active. The sharing of these dances often reveals new possibilities that lead to constructive change, helps us understand more about what we want, or how we block ourselves from getting what we want and need.

S U M M A R Y

In this class or series of classes, explore the issue of relationships through the metaphors of passive and active movements. Begin each class with a check-in, and a sensory aware-ness exercise that helps participants distinguish between tension and relaxation. These two qualities are often part of our ease or our difficulty in being passive or active, so being able to distinguish between the two will help participants embody the rest of the class material. Then, using a series of partnering scores, work with passive and active movements, alternating roles between leader and follower. Always switch roles when doing these scores so that participants can have the experience of playing both roles. It is important to leave time for drawing and a verbal check-in after each evolution of the material. This gives participants an opportunity to both share their personal experience and hear from their partners what was happening for them. As with all classes, practice active listening as participants share their experiences with one another.

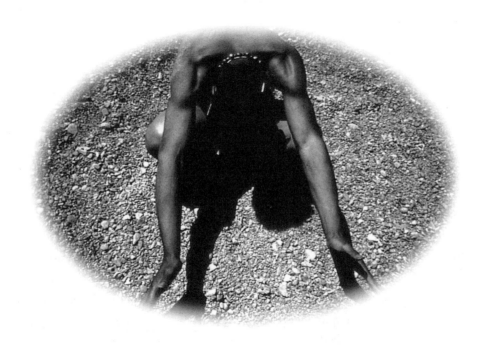

That suffering also which I showed to thee and the rest in the dance,
I will that it be called a mystery.

— HYMN OF JESUS, *Acts of St. John*

My intention in this session is to dance our prayers, to explore how, when, where, and why we pray, and to experience our relationship of prayer to healing. Take a moment to remember the last time you prayed. What was it like? Whom did you pray to? Why did you pray? When was the last time you danced your prayers? When I think of prayer many impressions rise up in me. I recall a lovely mythical story my friend Rabbi Brodie told me.

"In the beginning, God was everywhere. God occupied the entire cosmos. Then God wanted to create the world and fill it with all living things. So God had to make space. As she moved aside, she left sparks of her spirit drifting in the void. This was her spirit of goodness, mercy, compassion, forgiveness, and love. When she made vessels of all shapes for all living matter, these drifting sparks were contained in each vessel. As the people of the world began to live, these vessels became tarnished by the wars, cruelty, suffering, and human greed that allowed the earth to become polluted and for people to turn against each other. The sparks no longer shined through the vessels. Prayer is a way to once again illuminate the vessels so they will shine brightly and light up the whole world and all the creatures within her."

The following report from the book *The Cancer Puzzle* certainly affirms the value of prayer: "In one celebrated experiment, cardiologist Randolph Byrd at San Francisco General Hospital enlisted persons from across the United States to pray for roughly half of the 393 individuals admitted to the coronary care unit who either had actual heart attacks or severe chest pain. In this double-blind controlled experiment, neither the patients nor the physicians knew who was and was not being prayed for. Those for whom prayer was offered did better on several counts. There were fewer deaths; patients required less potent medication; and none required mechanical breathing support. This study is an example of how prayer can be tested clinically, much like a new medication or surgical procedure."

H O W   T O   B E G I N

The venue for this class could be anywhere, but be aware of how profoundly the environment can effect and influence the people in your class. Think of all the places that people have built for prayer—the great cathedrals, the eloquent monasteries, temples, synagogues, and elaborate mosques. Think also of simple and humble underground kivas built out of earth. I have been to gatherings for prayers in garages, dingy rooms in a slum district, outdoors in the wilderness, by the ocean, or around the table in my home. The point is: human beings can and do pray anywhere. Any venue can become a transformational space.

I encourage you to invest special consideration and care when preparing the space you will use for this session. Invite the participants to take part in creating a meaningful space. Incorporate the preparation of the space into this session. Inform the participants the week before that this session will be for prayer and discuss their ideas about the space, and about how they wish to pray. Perhaps people will bring sacred objects or other personal things. They may all decide to dress in a certain way. They may want to build an altar or bring cloth or something to mark the four directions. If you open up the idea of preparing the environment, people will have a million ideas.

When people arrive, allow time for them to alter the space and prepare it for the prayer session. Do a circle check-in. After the check-in when you feel the mood of the group, you can decide whether to begin the sensory awareness with the breath or the pulse. Here's a short sensory awareness exercise that incorporates both. We need sufficient time to develop the theme of the session, so I suggest that you keep this part brief.

S E N S O R Y   A W A R E N E S S

1. Find a place on the floor to stand.

2. Sense the weight of your body spreading along the soles of your feet. Shift your weight from front to back, and side to side.

3. Breathe out and imagine your weight dropping into the bottom of your feet and moving three feet past them into the earth. Take a long pause. Imagining the movement beginning at the bottom of your feet, let your elbows, lower arms, hands, and fingers reach to the sky. Then drop your arms.

4. Drop your head, letting your chin rest on your chest with your head close to your body. Continue dropping your head and let out a sigh as you release it. Become aware of the stretch in the back of your neck. Breathe deeply and relax. Give the weight of your head over to gravity and begin to slowly move down towards the ground. In sequence, flex one vertebra after the other. Emphasize the exhalation and sigh each time you breathe out.

5. When your head drops as far as your pelvis, flex your knees, and allow your arms to dangle in front of you.

6. Sense your spine from your tail bone to the top of your neck.

7. Reverse this movement, bringing your head back to an upright position. Move slowly, vertebra by vertebra. Place an accent on your inhalation, and become aware of a growing sense of lightness in your spine.

8. Repeat this same movement with a partner. One partner stands behind the other, guiding the unfolding of your partner's spine by touching one vertebra after the other. Imagine the vertebrae as the keys on a piano and your partner sliding up and down the scales, touching each note in sequence. Be that precise.

9. When you reach an upright position, bring your attention to the top of your head, and let your energy continue rising up to the sky above you.

10. Switch roles.

This sensory awareness exercise also evokes sensations and movements that will be useful resources for the dances we will eventually create during this class session. This is a good example of the congruency between movement and feelings. This "uplifting" movement with the spine usually creates an "uplifted" feeling in the participants.

M O V E M E N T   R E S O U R C E S

1. By yourself, repeat the same movement as in the previous exercise, and this time shift your awareness to the feeling evoked by the movement.

2   Stop and explore the feelings that arise in different places along your spine.

3. Do your feelings change as you rise? How? Take your time. Do they change when you are bent over?

4. Linger in any one of these moments and explore your movements and feelings.

5. Experiment with at least five different positions.

6. Pay attention to the connections between your movement and your feelings. Do any images come to you?

7. Add sounds. Add words. Add arm gestures.

8. Go all the way to the ground if your movement leads you there. Go forward and backward or in other directions in space if the movement and feelings take you there.

9. Contract and expand your movements using different degrees of force.

Follow the group and judge the amount of time to spend on this by the degree of their involvement. If you play music, avoid choosing anything people would have strong associations with, such as the Ave Maria or some of Bach's loftier compositions. The music is often so familiar that there is a danger that participants will follow the vivid tone of the music rather then their own true impulses. After this I suggest you take a break. You have some options here. Since this material is very inwardly focused and powerful, you may want to suggest that participants remain quiet during the break, write in their journals, or talk about their experiences with another person. Suggest that they sustain the mood of the class during their break.

THE PULSE

When the group returns, introduce improvising with a pulsing movement for two reasons: to energize the body, and to show participants that exhilarating movements carry as much potential for prayer as inwardly focused, quiet ones do.

1. Make yourselves comfortable and close your eyes. Take a few moments to connect with your breath and clear your mind.

2. Allow an image to emerge from this quiet space. It could arise from one of many different sources: a tilt of your head or the shape of your hand or the feeling of the "divine spark" inside you. Whom are you praying to? What are you praying for? Out of your quietness an image will come to you.

3. Draw your image.

4. Write a poem, a chant, a single word, or a sentence.

5. Share what you have created with another person.

DANCING OUR PRAYERS

We are ready now to do our dances. Ask the group if they would like the support of music or if they find music distracting. Go either way. Mostly people ask for the support of the music. Give them all the time they need. Encourage the dancers to be open to any outcome, no matter how different it might be from what they imagined. This dance can take between ten and twenty minutes. One group that had become very close did individual prayer dances and then naturally came together into small groups and finally into one large group to dance their collective prayer.

After we dance together, share your drawings and your experiences. Dennis's drawing had "gratitude" written under it. Dennis was having a very rough time with his illness. His cancer had spread throughout his body. He is the young father of two little boys. In spite of so much suffering, he still found gratitude. His drawing was of a round ball of vibrant orange and yellow colors; his dance was gentle and reverent. Each person's

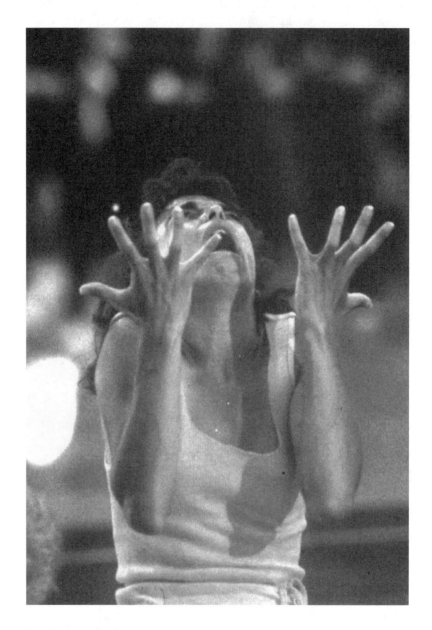

Imploring a higher power—

"Where can I turn for help? Why have you forsaken me."

image will be highly original, as are the many meanings and ways in which we dance, yet they all will carry the common thread of a deep sense of reverence and a passionate spirit. Structure and supporting resources for the group to work with can be minimal in this session because the need for prayer is so great that most people will find it easy to plunge right into the core of this material.

After you have done your prayer dances, and without talking, dismantle the altar you have created together, and return the room to its original state. Let this activity be a reminder of your prayer as well. In closing,

1. Form a circle and sit down. Hold hands, and close your eyes.
2. As you breathe out, begin to make a soft vocal sound.

3. Listen to each other and blend your sounds.

4. Allow the sound to develop and express how you feel as a group.

Often this kind of song will take some time to complete itself. Give it space to evolve in its own time. When it is finished, silently touch the earth, and reach your arms and chest toward the sky. If anyone needs special attention place them in the center of your circle. You can do this during the song so they can receive the vibrations of the group sound.

In the past, I have been shy in talking about this special kind of prayer for fear that by naming the sacred it would go away. Prayer seemed intangible to me; something I could not analyze as I could other things. It may be that in facing my own mortality, first when struck with cancer and now again as an elder, I can accept the awesome mystery of life and death and name it. You can too, without waiting so long.

SUMMARY

Prepare the environment for prayer. Allow the participants to help create a specific environment for this session. Introduce a sensory awareness exercise that focuses on the rising and falling of the spine. Then connect this movement to the feelings, emotions, and images that arise while you do this. This is the movement resource for the prayer dance. Make a drawing after doing this exercise and share it with a partner. Then allow the participants to dance their prayers. They can choose whether they wish to be accompanied by music or not. If the group chooses to dance together, encourage this. Close this session with a non-verbal check-out, during which chanting and singing will be appropriate for everyone.

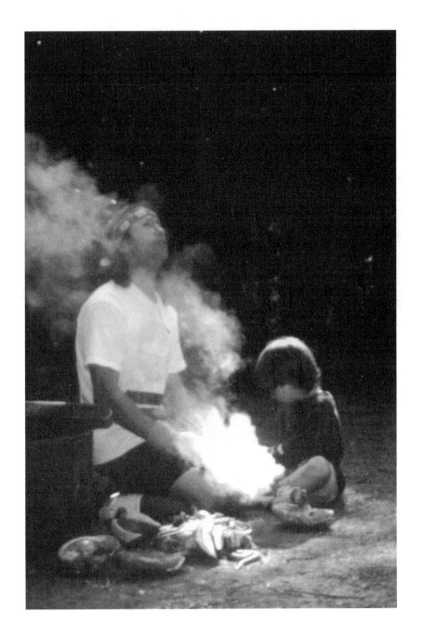

Preparing the environment for prayer.

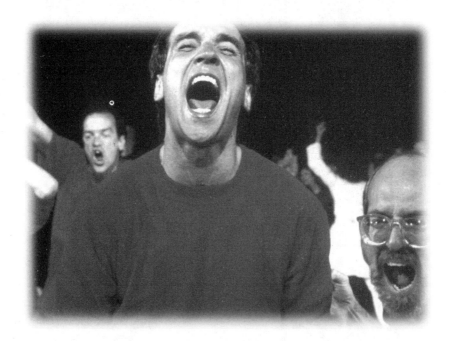

OUT OF MY BLOOD, MY BODY, MY MIND,

OUT, OUT, OUT!

The DNA of each of our cells carries a highly individualized signature, a "logo" of our unique embodied experience. Our immune system recognizes this DNA logo and consumes any cell that doesn't carry it, protecting our body from infection and illness. The immune system is like a catfish, a bottom feeder, sifting sand through its gills, constantly sorting waste from food. Catfish are vigilant; they never sleep. They make rapid and accurate decisions regarding the maintenance of their environment. Like a catfish, a healthy immune system keeps watch out for "predators", foreign matter in the blood that doesn't belong there. In this way, the immune system defends our identity on the cellular level. When cancerous cells grow in the body, however, the immune system becomes comprised and the vital functions of the body start to break down.

WHAT IS CANCER?

Cellular biology has revealed that cancerous cells are weak and confused cells. Rather than the strong ravaging predator we sometimes imagine, a cancer cell contains the incorrect genetic information which renders it incapable of performing its intended function. This incorrect genetic information arises due to exposure to harnful substances, chemicals, or damage by other external causes. And sometimes the body, which produces billions and billions of cells, creates an imperfect one. If a cell with incorrect genetic information begins to reproduce, then a tumor (or mass) of these cells begins to form. Ordinarily, the immune system, the body's natural defenses, recognizes and destroys these cells. But when malignant cancer cells grow, sufficient cellular changes take place, which makes it possible for them to reproduce quickly and attach to healthy cells throughout the body. When we are well, these cells "communicate" with one another. Malignant cells, however, do not respond to the communications from the healthy cells around them, and begin to reproduce recklessly. This rapid reproduction affects the immune system and the healthy function of other parts of the body. The malignant cancer cells compromise the normally vigilant immune system. The faulty cells of the tumor may begin to block proper functioning of the body organs, either by expanding and putting pressue on healthy organs, or by replacing healthy cells with malignant cells. In severe forms of cancer, malignant cells break off from the original mass and travel to other parts of the body, where they begin to reproduce and form new tumors. This is called "metastasis."

The immune system is a natural defense system built into the body for eliminating cancer or any other foreign cells that threaten our health. We need our immune systems to be strong and adaptable. This session is about one way in which we can connect and identify with this vital physical system. It has been discovered by doctors and other health practitioners that a conscious relationship to the immune system actually enhances and, to a great degree, determines its strength. We already have a relationship with this system on a deep and unconscious level; in this session, we will try to enhance this existing relationship through expressive movement and imagery.

There is a vast amount of important new information available about the immune system from the scientific community, which is being updated by the minute. There are many articles and books written on this subject that can provide you with exciting and useful information. I encourage you to do your own research if you are interested in more specific details about the immune system. Of great interest to the work of dance as a healing art are the connections being made between emotions and attitudes and their effects on the activities of the immune system.

When the immune system goes into action, each cell has a different function, operating as part of a remarkably organized team. In this session, we will dramatize the way the immune system operates and then find an image for it that will deepen our subjective experience of this invisible, physical reality taking place continuously in our bodies. But first, we do our usual check-in, followed by sensory awareness and movement resource exercises.

SENSORY AWARENESS - RELAX AND ENERGIZE

1. Shake your hands, your legs and your arms. Focus on your sensations.

2. Jump or wiggle and shake yourself like a rag doll. Feel your bones and joints.

3. While you are jumping and shaking, make sounds connected to your movements.

4. Continue to explore the connection between movement and sound until you are ready to stop and catch your breath.

5. Stretch and collapse. Breathe out with a loud breathy sound.

WORKING TOGETHER

Any game structure that acts as an energizer and promotes teamwork is appropriate at this point. Red Light! Green Light!, a popular children's game, generates alertness, while Tug-of-War will mobilize strength and determination. You may have a favorite game you'd like to use.

TUG-OF-WAR

1. Put one person on either end of the rope. Have each person pull in the opposite direction. Use your voice as you pull and sense your whole body mobilizing itself.

2. Gradually add people to either end of the rope to make this into a team exercise. If there are some people who do not have the physical strength to do these movements, they can urge their teammates to victory by shouting or cheering.

After you have finished with this game, I suggest this next exercise to generate movement resources.

MOVEMENT RESOURCES

1. Begin to walk through the space, making eye contact with everyone else.

2. Walk in the spaces between other people.

3. Walk and look around you.

4. Walk and patrol the room.

5. Roam around and look around you.

6. Walk with urgency and alertness, as if you were on the lookout for danger.

7. Place a large pillow or some type of large soft object on the floor. This will represent a group of cancer cells.

8. One by one, each person approaches this group of cancer cells, and each in her own way uses movement and sound to attack, eliminate, transform, destroy, or slaughter them. Call upon whatever strategy you have for this.

9. Let your movements express how you feel about your cancer cells. Use your voice. Be as real and convincing as you can with whatever approach you choose.

Doing this exercise will lead invariably to conversations about our attitude towards the cancer cells. The stance we take as we perform these exercises also reveals how determined and committed we are to eliminating or destroying the cancer cells, and the strategies we employ to do so. The leader should encourage and help each participant in the effective execution of the movements. Some people resist attacking their cancer cells, and instead want to treat them as if they were friends who had gone astray. Some people may want to transform them through love. You will hear all sorts of attitudes. Whatever your personal opinion is about how to face cancer, it is your responsibility as the leader to give each person an opportunity to express fully and with conviction her own response to the cancer cells and to the illness.

In this crisis of healing, each person has to find her own way back to health. Seeing what other people do may affect someone's attitudes and possibly influence or even open up new options, but there are certain ideas you may want to keep in mind and share with your class. Remind participants that it is nature's way to destroy cells that threaten the survival of the body and that this process is going on in each person's body right now. People often place a moral judgment on the notion of "killing" the cell. We can substitute the word "kill" and replace it with "eliminate," "transform," "flush out," etc. We are not referring to destruction in some wanton, immoral way. But we are talking about survival. The bottom line question that comes up is this: What are you willing to do to save your life? Under what circumstances are you willing to do it?

Peggy Rogers told me a stunning story that illustrates this point; a Buddhist monk allowed himself to die of cancer because he believed that if the cancer cell in his body wanted to live, he would let it live. He would not kill anything, not even a cancer cell that would kill him. He made no attempt to save his life. Whereas a nun he knew had cancer and with his blessing, availed herself of every treatment. The lesson of this story is that we each must understand for ourselves what we are willing to do to survive, the nature of our own will to live, and the form and actions this takes in our lives.

In this class session, I always hand out a copy of the description of the immune system as prepared by the Cancer Support and Education Center. This description is printed at the end of this chapter. Feel free to copy it and give it to the participants in your class. You can use it as a resource for developing a class session, or as a plan for your approach to the drama of the immune system. Look at this chart before you attempt to work out your scores. Dancing this "drama" will be the core experience of this session.

THE IMMUNE SYSTEM DRAMA

The idea of this section of class is to act out the drama of the immune system in relation to the cancer cells. The basic narrative is as follows. The cells in the immune system are always on the alert, pacing and patrolling for any possible cancer cells lurking around. The cancer cells have broken ties with the harmony of the system of normal cells. They are out of control, wild, and confused. They find an opening in the defenses of the immune system and begin to invade. The immune system immediately goes to work. The body's alarm is sounded, and all the defensive cells rush to the site of the invasion. The healthy immune system destroys, outwits, out maneuvers, defeats, slaughters, eliminates, transforms, convinces, purifies, and expels the cancer cells. The cancer cells die, and the host organism is returned to health.

Form two groups. Ask everyone to select a cell they would like to role-play. Refer to the handout at the end of this chapter for a description of these resources. Each person should become familiar with the characteristics of the cell they will act out. Work together as a team and have a good time deciding how you will act out this drama! Each group should discuss ideas, choose roles, and invent a strategy. Participants can use

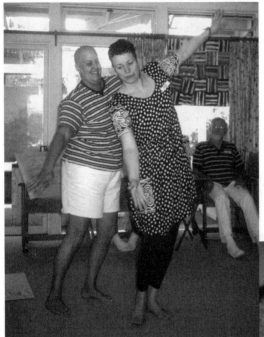

Dancing in pairs, our hearts are
relieved of their burdens.

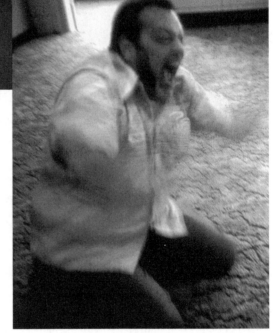

Shouting at his cancer cells:
"I will rip you to shreds."

sounds, words, props, or anything they wish to characterize their parts. The teacher can act as facilitator/director. Your own enthusiasm for this process will inspire the group. Plan that each group will perform for the other. Before a group begins, do a physical preparation to energize the body. One group should perform their dance while the other supports them however they can. Then reverse roles, so everyone gets a chance to perform and witness. In addition, I suggest that you do it twice, and have people shift roles so that everyone gets to be a cancer cell, and a cell in the immune system. Make sure that all the cells are represented in each group. There can be more then one person playing a cell.

The cancer cells need to be dealt with quite differently in movement than the cells of the immune system. Performers who want to be the cancer cells may want to take on movements that are stupid, out of control and confused. I suggest that very little force or vigor is given to the cancer cells. Be sensitive to yourself when acting out this role. Avoid becoming attached to it. Sometimes it is useful to have an object, rather than a person, represent the cancer cell. This way, no one has to face the aggressive energy directed at the cancer cell. On the other hand, it can also be of great benefit to act out the death of the cell.

I have seen people in the role of the cancer cell being unwilling to die or be transformed. Does this mean they are holding on to their illness for some unconscious reason? Or are they just unable to relax and let go? Perhaps there is a habit blocking the physical sensation of letting go. In this case, you can help the person rediscover that movement option. This is an example of the feedback process between movement and feelings. When you cannot access a particular movement, you will not be able to experience the matching feelings, and vice versa. As you can imagine, this can have far-reaching implications for our attitudes. If the attitudes are destructive, we have an opportunity to change them by finding movements that are positive.

VISUALIZATION AND
GROUP DANCE

After the immune system dance, take a break and prepare for the next step in the process. It is time now to find a way to personalize the immune system through the use of visualization. Ask participants to find a place to rest quietly and close their eyes.

1. Take a few deep breaths.

2. Allow an image to enter your mind's eye that represents a cell in the immune system. Take your time. The image can be a creature or a fantasy or anything that represents a cell that can effectively destroy, eliminate, or transform your cancer cells.

3. See it very clearly. How will it do its job for you? What does it look like? What does it say? What sounds does it make? How does it move?

4. Have a dialogue with it. Ask how it will do its job. Be precise and thorough, and demand the very best strategy.

5. When you are ready, make a drawing of your image.

6. Reinforce this drawing by emphasizing the parts that are most important for the cell to do its job. Draw thicker lines, or use more intense colors. Encourage participants to do more with their drawings.

7. When the drawings are finished, write down a plan for eliminating your cancer cells. This is a crucial part of the process and needs to be given time and attention. Give this image words to say to your cancer cells.

8. Share your drawing and writing with a partner.

9. Dance your drawing with your partner supporting you in any way you choose. She can reinforce your dance with the words you have written.

10. Change roles.

11. Discuss with each other the message of this visualization, and how it affects your life.

It is amazing to see all the different images people find for their immune system. Here are just a few examples: One woman saw a spiral vacuum cleaner in radiant pastel colors sucking up all the cancer cells. As they pass through the vacuum cleaner, they are transformed into white light. Another saw a vicious, menacing snake darting with the speed of lightning, striking the cancer cells with its electric tongue and instantly killing them. A third participant imagined a lion patrolling its territory and smelling the cancer cells from any distance, pouncing on them and shredding them to pieces. An ancient turtle living at the bottom of the ocean who knows when cancer cells are there was imagined by someone else. The turtle calmly floats to the top, sticking its head out and plucking the cancer cells methodically from the sea, never missing one. An unusual image came from a women who imagined a skunk. She said this skunk could simply and elegantly lift its tail and spray. The intense odor suffocated the cancer cells, rendering them helpless.

There is a certain mystery in these images. Where they come from is beyond analysis. It is enough to know that they are to be trusted and that each person has a reason for the image they have found. Suggest that each person give a name to her image, call on it each day, and practice using it for protection. When we continue to use images in this manner, they grow in clarity and strength, and the healing strategies we have uncovered through this image will become more effective. Try it. Include a meditation on this image as a daily practice. The next week, ask for a report on how people used their images.

CHECK-OUT

At check-out, sit in a circle and tell one another how and what you can do in your lives to keep your immune system healthy. Stand in a circle, raise all your arms in the air, and shout: POWER TO THE WHITE CELLS!

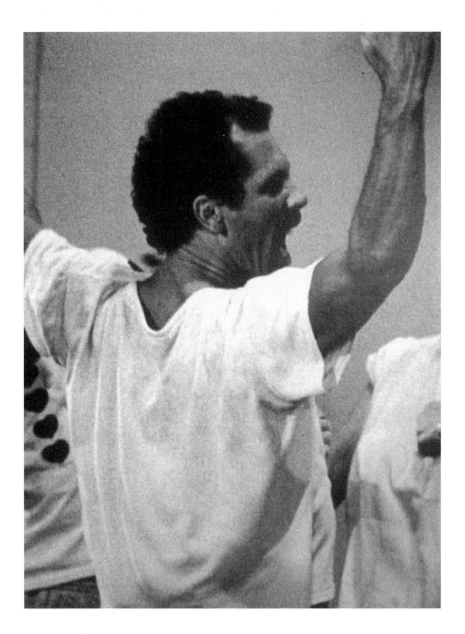

Power to the white cells.

SUMMARY

This class is serious fun and offers both subjective and objective information about the immune system. It is one of the most useful themes in this series because the directed use of the image of cancer cells can change people's relationship to their illness. After check-in and warming up through sensory awareness, generate movement resources and then move into the game of acting out the drama of the immune system. Each participant should play a different role, and then switch roles so that they can experience both sides of the conflict. This dramatization gives us insights about our attitudes toward our illness. Then do a visualization to discover an image of protection and a strategy for using it. Share this information in partners, and then with the whole group.

DESCRIPTION OF THE IMMUNE SYSTEM

HELPER T-CELL sounds alarm to arouse the whole immune system, and boosts the aggressiveness of the other white cells. It does this by releasing a chemical message.

NATURAL KILLER CELL, a "free spirit," constantly roaming on patrol. Detects the presence of tumors or virus-infected cells. Hunts them down and destroys them by injecting poison into them. Can act independently of Helper T-Cell input.

KILLER T-CELL, also on patrol, hunts own cancerous and virus-infected cells and kills them by injecting poison. Relies on Helper T-Cells for information. Travels where needed.

B-CELL hovers around the lymph nodes. Produces antibodies (immunoglobulins). The antibodies attach themselves to viruses and inactivate them.

MACROPHAGE is the "great eater." Engulfs and destroys invaders. Eats debris and diseased tissue. Signals the presence of invaders to the other immune cells. Constantly roams on patrol.

SUPPRESSER T-CELL dampens or slows down vigilance to return to normal activity of the other white cells after the battle is over. Allows the level of vigilance to return to normal.

QUALITIES OF THE IMMUNE SYSTEM

COMMON ROOTS: Each white cell is born in the bone marrow. About half of them migrate to the thymus to become T-Cells. The other half become Macrophages, B-Cells, or Natural Killer Cells. Nerve endings reach into the bone marrow and thymus, forming one pathway of communication from the brain to the organs of the immune system.

REDUNDANCY: There are "compensatory mechanisms" built into the immune system. This means there is overlap between the functions of various types of white cells.

This diversity helps the system compensate when certain parts are not working properly. For example, long term AIDS survivors may have poor T-Cell function, but high Natural Killer Cell function.

INTELLIGENCE: All the white cells have senses and intelligence. They literally think and communicate with each other. They receive information from the brain also, by way of neuropeptides being released by the brain in response to images, moods, and beliefs. Each cell carries a genetic image of how to do its work, and what health looks like.

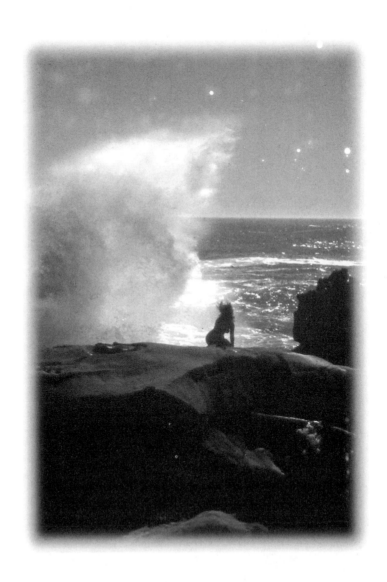

Nature is but another name for health

and seasons are but different states of health.

HENRY DAVID THOREAU, *Journal, August 23, 1853*

May all I say and all I think be in harmony with trees

God within me God beyond me, maker of the trees.

CHINOOK PSALTER

The intention of this session is to make direct contact with nature, and specifically, to connect with a tree. This same lesson plan could be applied to any element in the natural world—a stone, a rock, a flower, a river, sand, and so forth. In this session we will actually be outdoors physically touching a part of the natural world, but it is also possible to use these materials as a visualization, if an appropriate natural environment is not available. Ideally, however, the location of this session is outdoors in a grove of redwood or other trees. The next chapter will give you more information about how to access the natural world through visualizations, no matter where you are.

We are all part of a bigger body, and that bigger body is nature herself. We are water, metal, earth, and air. We are nature, not separate from it. Our skin is an envelope holding part of our nature within; it forms a boundary between us and the outer world, but that outer world is also part of us, and we are part of it. It is an illusion of the mind that the inner and outer landscapes are separate. I believe that the inner and outer landscapes are one. By connecting with this larger body, we can find a life-giving support that is often neglected and denied in our industrialized culture. A group of very wise women in their nineties were presiding on a panel. When they were asked, "Where do you find your strength?" each one included nature as a great strength-giver in their lives. As an elder myself, I can say that I find tremendous peace when I am close to the vital sources of the natural world. All my worries, responsibilities, and obligations fade away as I become at one with what is around me. Simply walking in the woods, or by the ocean, does wonders to restore the life force.

The focus of this class is to heighten our awareness of the natural world and to experience how this awareness can support our healing. We begin again with a circle check-in. Imagine that the check-in is filled with stories of pain, fatigue, doubt, and depression. There is a low mood in the group. We all listen to each other respectfully without trying to change the way anyone is feeling. What do you do when your group is feeling low? You move. The following is an example of how you might pick up on the needs of the group through movement.

SENSORY AWARENESS

This exercise needs to be leisurely. Take plenty of time. The touching and stroking is comforting and keeps our attention on waking up our senses.

1. Make a small circle, and close your eyes.

2. Place your hands on your chest. Inhale and fill your hands with your breath. Hold your breath. Then breathe out and stroke your chest, slowly.

3. Repeat the action of breathing into your hands through your chest, holding your breath, exhaling, and stroking your chest.

4. Vary the parts of your body that you stroke. With your attention, follow the stroking sensation in your arms, down to your belly, and along your sides. Take your time.

5. Let the strokes follow the contours of your body until you have stroked your whole body, including your face and scalp. What sensations are you aware of now?

6. Clap your hands lightly on your chest as if it were a drum. Turn to a friend next to you and begin to lightly tap her back.

7. Experiment with clapping, tapping, and brushing each other. When you are done, switch partners and play with someone else.

This activity invariably will take you out of your head and into your body. This exercise generally has an immediate effect. It will help you become more present in your body, and your worries and fears will begin to be suspended, if only for this moment. We are ready to move on to the theme of this session.

MOVEMENT EXPLORATION

We identify intuitively with trees through our bodies. A tree has a trunk like the trunk of our body; it has limbs as we do; it has four directions—front, back, side, and side— and together these directions make a round shape. A tree stands vertically and when it falls, it lies horizontally. There are other associations with trees that are more emotional and symbolic. Here is a list generated in one of my class sessions: strength; childhood; freedom; comfort; power; inner parent/father; earth/sky connection; communication.

1. Start with movements relating to the trunk of your body and the spine. Explore the ways your arms and legs come out of and relate to your trunk.

2. Rise to a standing position. Be aware of the earth and the sky in this activity of rising.

3. Look around at the trees and explore arm movements suggested by the limbs of trees; hands and fingers from the leaves; body shapes from the trunk, grounding in the feet and legs from the roots. Do this slowly and notice the qualities and feelings connected to your movements.

If you are working in a different environment such as the ocean, you would want your movement explorations to pertain to the motion of the waves and the wind, rather than the shapes of trees. Accommodate your movement resources to the environment where you work.

BLINDFOLD WALK

After the movement exploration, return to a sensory awareness exercise by taking a blindfold walk.

The tree is in you. You are in the tree.

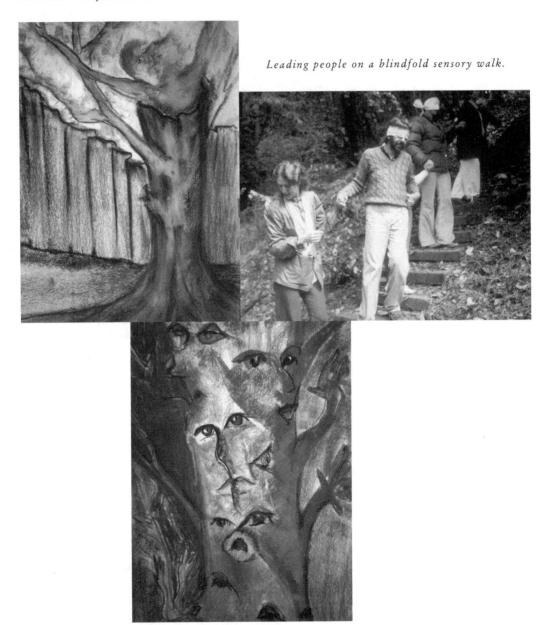

Leading people on a blindfold sensory walk.

"Did you know that trees talk? Well, they do. They talk to each other, and they talk to you if you listen. I have learned a lot from trees about my healing."

1. Stand behind one another in a line, and hold a twig or branch connecting each person to the person in front of her, avoiding the human touch which you would have if you held hands.

2. The leader of the line has her eyes open and leads the group through a wooded area (or whatever environment you are in).

This simple activity is a powerful experience. No matter how many times you may have done this, it remains equally powerful. Although we are in a procession, we are not going anywhere. We are already there; each step is its own experience. The array of sensations and feelings accompanying this walk can be incredibly rich. The leader can help participants distinguish between senses by stopping the walk at different intervals and asking them to focus on listening, smelling, touching, or tasting their environment. There is hardly a more concentrated method of kinesthetic sensing than moving with eyes closed and blocking out our most familiar sense—the sense of sight.

FINDING YOUR TREE

Once you arrive in the site where you will be working, participants should remove their blindfolds, and begin a more personal journey through the environment.

1. Find a tree that calls to you and go to it.

2. Make physical contact with the tree, using different parts of your body. Touch the tree with your hands, face, chest, belly, back, front of pelvis, back of pelvis, thighs, feet, and legs. Lean into the tree. Embrace the tree. Stay in contact with the tree for at least ten minutes. It takes time to engage all of your senses in this contact.

3. Pay attention to feelings, emotions, and images stimulated by your contact with the tree.

DANCING YOUR TREE

1. Dance with your tree. Find yourself in relationship to it. The tree is in you; you are in the tree.

2. Find a way to close this dance.

3. Draw your tree and write about your experience.

People identify with nature by projecting themselves into its forms—in this instance, the form of a tree. From this process, we can obtain rich insights and meaningful connections to our life needs. Here are some of the things people saw and felt after this experience. One participant saw all the trees in the grove connected to one another in a deep and complex way. The tree became a symbol for community and the need to live in community in order to heal. Another participant saw the whole process of life, youth, and death in her tree. She saw the wounding and the healing, and experienced the totality of a being moving from one state to another over time. Another saw the tree as endless, a home that offered strength, safety, support, and reliable partnership. "It's OK to ask for support," her tree said.

One participant had a dialogue with her tree, as follows:

ME: Dear tree, how's it feel to be dead?

TREE: That's too obvious. Look at those green shoots up on top. Each one a new tree. Who says I'm dead?

ME: But you're burnt to a crisp!

TREE: The flames were so gorgeous I burned in ecstasy, the energy so translucent, so insistent. Silly sister, you don't know very much!

ME: Am I your sister? I thought I was your daughter.

TREE: How presumptuous of you. Next to me, what are you? You're my little squirrel, my June bug, my weevil. You're a leaf torn from a neighbor, balancing on my charred rim.

ME: I want to stay here with you. What do you think?

TREE: Stop! You make me chortle down deep somewhere. Lord, almighty, my roots are still alive!

After this dialogue, she described her dance with the tree.

It was getting to be evening, the light was soft under the circle of big trees.
I began to dance the birth of my own tree. I grew taller and taller, opening limb
by limb, slowly, meeting the breeze and swaying, until I was a full-grown
redwood, standing so tall, reaching up into the universe. Then I imagined the
flames coming through the forest. I could hear them crackling. Finally
they reached me. I writhed in anguish, my branches curling and breaking and
falling, until I was stripped bare. Then I got smaller and smaller until I
was a charred stump. I huddled there, waiting for the first drops of rain to fall
on me. It felt ancient and magical to move that way as the light turned
gold-gray and then blue-gray and
the day dissolved. The silence welcomed
and held me.

Finally Anna asked us to complete our dances and sit in a circle. We talked
about our drawings and our dances. I felt a wholeness, an expansion and large
relaxation, a sense of being deeply part of life and sufficient in it. Anna said to
me after my dance: "Well, you did the whole life cycle, didn't you? Indeed.
I grew as the tree, opened to life, stood tall and proud, met the fire and was
eaten by it, fell back dead and waited, almost peacefully, for the rain to
revive me, and the new life to fall on my charred body, take root, and spring
up as a new tree. Now I feel a profound satiety and sense of rightness, my
body opened and larger somehow, my mind pleased and listening, attending
to everything.

— *Written by* S A N D Y   B O U C H E R

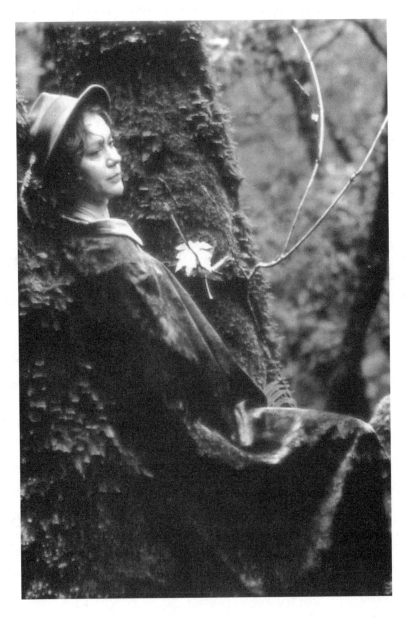

Making contact with a tree.

CLOSURE

For your closure, sit in a circle. Have a collection of seven stones that can fit into the palm of your hand. One by one, let each person place them in a configuration in the center of the circle. Read the message of the stones. This activity has some of the same possibilities as sand-tray play, and it always yields creative and insightful results. This is akin to the ancient Chinese divination system of the I Ching, in which you throw yarrow sticks to the ground, and read their symbolic message. You can do this just as well with sticks or leaves. Then, touch the earth, stand, and reach toward the sky in silence. Leave each other in this reverent manner.

SUMMARY

In this class, we refer to nature as a healer and use the outdoor environment as a way to teach us something about ourselves. Beginning with a check-in and a sensory warm-up, the material of the day concerns the embodiment of a principle of nature. Take the participants on a blindfold walk to increase their kinesthetic sensitivity and then allow them to make contact with an element in nature, specifically a tree. Because there is a deep and intuitive resonance between the human and the natural world, participants will find ways of communicating with the trees that are beyond language or specific conscious understanding. Time to dance with the trees, write about the trees, and draw the trees will deepen their understanding of their relationship to the nature within themselves.

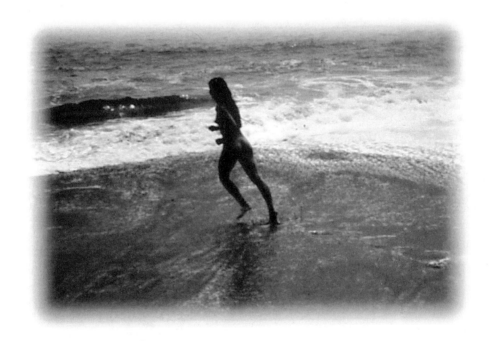

I SAW MYSELF RUNNING BY THE SEA,

FEELING THE SUN ON MY BACK,

FEELING WELL, AND FREE.

Teaching in a situation where people are facing a life-threatening illness requires a totally different attitude than teaching a traditional dance class. With this work, the teacher needs to have a backlog of resources to meet the immediate needs of the participants, rather than being attached to a more logical lesson plan that might relate to what you did the week before, or what you plan to do the week after. It doesn't always work this way—what prevails is the condition the participants are in when they come to you.

Here is an example. I had been working on a series of lessons about relationships to family and friends. I had carefully designed a lesson continuing on this theme. During the check-in, each person reported on a very immediate and intense situation. One person's voice was quivering as she told us that this was the anniversary of her husband's death and that she had just gotten news that her husband's father had died. Her own mother and father had died that year. She was feeling very vulnerable. Another person brought her mother to class, a 77-year-old woman with a debilitating case of Parkinson's disease, who was recently diagnosed with terminal cancer and was undergoing chemotherapy. I was particularly touched by the relationship between the mother and the daughter because the daughter had studied dance with me starting at the age of four, and I remember distinctly when her mother brought her to class she said to her daughter, "You don't have to do anything, but you do have to be here." Her daughter, who is now in her late forties, turned to her mother and said, "Mother, you don't have to do anything, but you do have to be here." Another woman complained of excruciating pain in her back. She has chronic fatigue syndrome, chronic pain, and struggles with cancer. She was feeling rotten. Continuing around the circle, everyone shared a sense of deep depression and low energy.

This kind of situation is not unusual, and for this reason, I want to suggest how you might choose to deal with this. Have everybody leave their chairs and lie on the floor. Lying on the floor is more relaxing than standing or sitting. When lying down, our bodies are given full support through the floor. This can be comforting, and relaxing. The next step is to choose an entry point to the body. There are four places to begin: sensation, movement, feelings, or images. Because people were depressed and in pain, their physical bodies were in many ways unavailable to them. When this happens, taking people into the realm of images often facilitates a connection to the body through a more spiritual dimension.

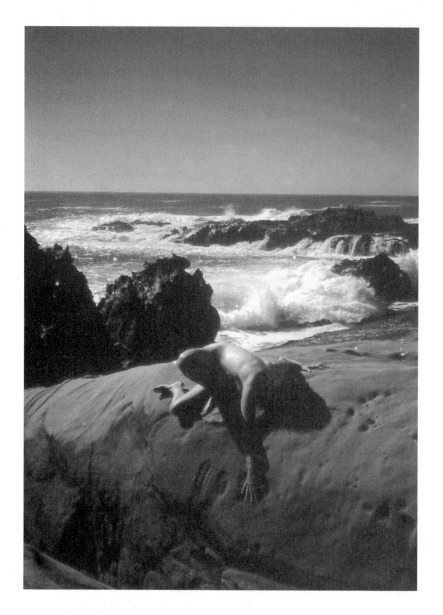

The body in harmony with nature.
   Returning to the source inspires spiritual strength.

Use a guided image focusing on the ocean, the sky, and the sun. These images can bring us in touch with our innate relationship to the larger life force. When people are in pain, it is often helpful for them to be able to identify with the larger body of nature of which they are intrinsically a part. You will find that participants can feel the nature inside their bodies, of which they are sometimes unaware. Being reminded of this will be of benefit to them. It is valuable for them to discover their relationship to nature as an available resource in their healing. As you read the following material, I want to remind you that it is more important for you to understand the principles of this meditation than it is to learn this specific one. You can always make up your own meditations to suit the needs of the participants.

Here is the guided image:

"Allow yourselves to be filled and infused with the expansive image of a vast blue sky. Feel its limitlessness, spaciousness, and clarity. Breathe deeply, inhaling this sense of freedom, and exhaling any sense of limitation. Let your mind dissolve. As the calm, open breath finds its own natural rhythm, begin to bring your attention to the center of your ribcage, inviting this expansive sky to accompany you there. This will help the ribcage to open, which in turn can change your feelings.

"Pause now, and begin to feel your way into the motion, sound, and texture of a deep green ocean. Let yourselves relax into the image, the power, and ancient timeless rhythm of her waves rising and falling, rising and falling, carrying you deeper and deeper into the organic pulse of your own life force, your own body. Travel with your breath down into your pelvis, sensing the ebb and flow of this image there. Restoring, healing, cleansing, renewing: the image itself and the place in which it lies will calm the rhythm of your breath. This image is designed to center and ground the body by bringing in new energy and life.

"Emerge gently and gradually from the depths of the ocean into a ray of sunlight as it filters down through the waves. Feel the warmth on your skin and allow it to penetrate right through flesh, muscle, fiber, releasing tension deep in the marrow of your bones. See the round yellow powerhouse extending its rays in all directions and draw it gradually into the center of your forehead, between your eyes, warming and evaporating, shining light into the space in which any negative thoughts might have taken hold. This image can relax tension in your jaws, and between your eyes, and clear your head."

The three colors suggested here —blue, green, and yellow—have been chosen quite consciously because they often show up in people's drawings as healing colors. The final image of the sun with its rays streaming down through the sky and deep into the ocean is symbolic of an integration of the three separate images.

When people's bodies have been altered—their breathing calmed, their eyelids still, their faces relaxed—continue to develop the images. "Bring in an image of your own into this landscape, something you imagine might be moving in the sky or in the ocean. Embody the image that you have created, just with your fingers. Gradually involve more parts of your body until you can move as freely as you choose, or with minimal movement. Do a drawing and writing piece after this."

Here are some examples of what came out of this image exercise:

Jean, the older woman with Parkinson's, drew an image of seaweed. She wrote, "I am the floating seaweed, moving freely in the water. No limits, no strain." She was able, through images, to experience herself moving in the comfort of water, effortlessly, with no strain. She had tapped into another aspect of her experience. She was smiling and asked to come back to class. She said this opened up a whole new world for her that she hadn't imagined possible. Jean died soon after this. Her family arranged a memorial, which was held at the ocean. Her daughter did a ritual with seaweed and ceremonially returned the seaweed to the water, as if it were a continuation of her mother's life and her spirit.

Sandra drew a picture of different kinds of active jungle animals. Some of them had blood dripping out of their mouths, and one was up in a tree for protection. They looked like they were on a hunt. She had drawn a line separating the animals from the sky, where there was a large blue cloud. She wrote, "Down below, all is struggle. They are stalking and eating each other. I am a cloud, floating above it." It seemed she had found some peace, detaching herself from her everyday struggles. If nothing more, she seemed to have found a momentary oasis from whatever difficulties she faced in her life.

Jane drew a big yellow sun, a vast blue sky, and a deep green ocean with rising and falling waves. The new image she put into the picture was a very large starfish almost the same size as the sun. It was a brilliant orange and red. She wrote, "Like a star, but just a fish. Seem to be moving slow, but a star seems that way too, and it goes all the way around the world in a day." This woman, suffering from chronic fatigue and constant pain, puts herself under constant pressure at work and at school. Perhaps her image was telling her she could slow down and still get around the world.

Ann, who was grieving the death of her husband and other members of her family, drew a fish, half in the water and half rising out of the water. She said it was a beautiful gold, sparkling fish and that it sparkled because it was wet. It was wild, free, sensuous. Then she went on to say, "I used to be afraid of them. I had nightmares that I was swimming with fish. One day, somebody dropped a dead goldfish in my lap as a joke and I panicked. Now, I love this fish." As she talked, she told us about an image of the fish coming out of the water and of her barbecuing and eating it. She was very pleased, laughed a lot, and kept saying, "This is amazing. I can't believe I love this fish."

In many traditions, the idea of eating a power animal is a way of embodying that power for yourself. I couldn't help but make this connection as I listened to her talk about her image. It is my point of view that making literary or intellectual connections of this sort is an interesting sideline for me personally, but I avoid sharing such information with the participants because I think it draws them away from their own physical and emotional experience and turns it into an intellectual exercise. Although I was interested in this connection, I did not want to divert this woman from her experience. Either she would find that power and transformation in her life, or she wouldn't, but I felt it wouldn't serve her to have projected this interpretation on her experience.

People left this session with a sense of hope. They were uplifted and awed by their own creativity and what they had revealed to themselves. There was another small spark ignited in their will to live, and the use of imagery led to very powerful and profound experiences. I believe that using imagery and writing in this instance was an immediate way to engage the participants because of all the senses, the visual and the auditory/cognitive senses are the most available to us in this culture. When we are shut down or in pain, it is very difficult to enter our bodies fully or with joy. Sometimes a back road to that more positive state of being is through imagery and visualizations.

SUMMARY

This lesson plan is an example of adapting to the specific and immediate needs of the participants. When people are in pain, choose the entry route to the sense of imagination. Much more so than movement or emotions, this sense is readily available, even when people are uncomfortable in their bodies. Lead the participants on a guided visualization that helps them connect to the larger principle of nature as it is located within their bodies. After the visualization, do a small dance, a drawing, and some writing. Then share what you have learned from the imagery exercise.

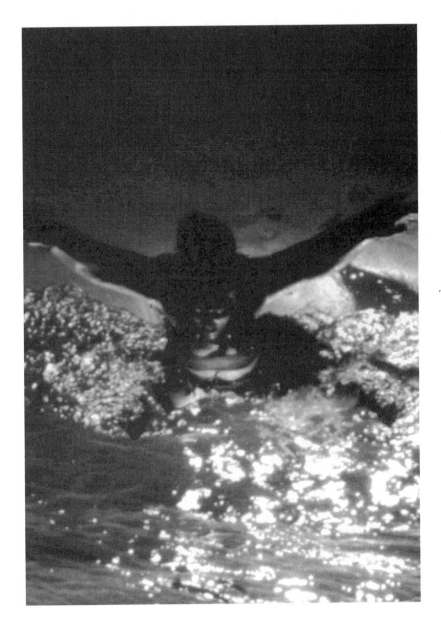

Creating an image focusing on water, sky, and the sun.

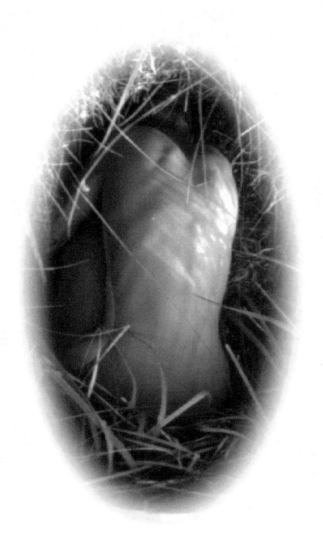

My spine, moving

Like kelp in the ocean's bed

— RACHEL KAPLAN

The intention in this session is to enable participants to fully experience a state of complete relaxation; practice witnessing their bodies in motion without the interference of the controlling mind; observe and appreciate the wonder of movement in a pure state; and to experience the interconnections between all parts of the body. Have you ever watched seaweed being moved by the tides, or a bird in flight when the wind allows it to soar, or the branches of a tree swaying with a gentle breeze or shaken by a violent wind? Remember the intricate patterns along the shore created by the incoming waves, or the jagged shapes of rocks created by millions of years of pounding ocean, or the clouds floating overhead carried by a wind current? Close your eyes and remember all the movement you experienced when witnessing these phenomena of nature. In this session, we will experience a principle akin to this as we allow our bodies to be moved by an outside force. We will witness in ourselves and our partner the pure beauty of ourselves in movement, much the way we can easily appreciate these patterns in nature. We do this through an activity called towelling.

Towelling is a name that was spontaneously given to a specific activity we do because bath-size towels are used as a prop for doing it. The activity could more aptly be called "river" because we duplicate some of the intrinsic flow of water in this exercise. Have enough towels on hand for each participant. A hand-size towel or a small bath towel will serve. We work in partners, using a towel in the central exercise of the class to avoid human touch, which might bring with it an expectation, a command, a comfort, or a correction. Obviously, I do not think human touch is bad, but in this experience, participants have a pure experience of their own movement without being concerned about anyone else.

C H E C K - I N

Start this class with a circle check-in. For a change, check-in with partners and have the partners report back to the larger circle. Choose a partner who is about your size because you will be moving each other's bodies in the following exercises. If it is at all possible, the ideal setup for this class would be to bring in assistants equal to the number of participants so that the participants could have the luxurious experience of being moved without having to switch roles and be someone else's mover. However, this is often not possible, but whenever you have assistants available to you, this is an excellent class for them to attend.

T O W E L L I N G

One person (A) will lie on the floor and relax. The other person (B) will create the outside force for A. A starts lying on the ground. B moves A with the towel.

1. Head: Put a towel under your partner's head. Slide it along the floor in different directions. Make a cradle out of it and lift the head out of gravity's pull. See how the whole body responds to this head movement. Rock and rotate the head. Slide the towel away and slowly brush it over the skin of your partner's face as if it were a gentle wind.

2. Arms: Place the towel at the elbow or wrist joint. Lift the arm and rock it back and forth in the shoulder socket. Move the arm up and then slowly drop it. Raise the arm above the head and watch its stretch affect the entire the ribcage. Cross the arm over the chest and draw it over the body until the shoulder blade opens, and further until the upper body rolls onto its side. Passive partner release arm to the ground. Let your arm be heavy. Carefully experiment with other ways you can move A's arms. Observe in detail how you are being an outer force moving your partner and how the movement operates in your body. Switch arms. When finished, brush towel over the arms.

3. Legs: Place the towel under the knee of one leg. Bend the knee and lift it. Move the leg in different directions. Carefully and slowly walk around your partner's body, holding the knee. Cross the leg over the body so the spine is in a rotation. Watch the

entire body respond to the movement of the leg. Again, experiment with movements you can do with the leg that affect the rest of the body. The legs tend to be heavy so do only what is comfortable for you. If you want to develop the movement, you can drag your partner across the floor and initiate a ripple effect throughout the body by zig-zagging.

4. Switch legs.

5. Brush the towel over the whole body as if it were the wind.

6. Break contact with your partner.

N A T U R E   D A N C E

After the towelling part of the exercise is complete, move into a "nature dance." The leader can play some soothing music at this time.

1. Partner A, move in your own way from that place of deep relaxation, and allow your movements to unfold according to your body's natural response to the towelling.

3. Partner B observe partner's dance. This might take five minutes or longer. Allow for this.

4. When ready, switch roles. Repeat the towelling part of the exercise. You might want to avoid talking and keep the whole exercise on the non-verbal level. Partner A now moves partner B in ways you particularly liked.

5. This time, after the towelling is complete, rather than observing your partner after you break contact with the towel, join in her dance, and maintain a state of relaxation.

When both people have done the exercise, come together and sit back to back and rest. What are the images, words, and feelings that arise? Stay in this relaxed state and let your mind flow without any pressure. When you are ready, draw an image of your movement experience. After drawing, free associate with words. When writing, use different colored crayons if you wish. Keep your words connected to your movements. Use the words you wrote to create a poem. Share your poem and drawing with your partner. Finish this exercise by sharing your experiences with the large group.

Here are two of the poems generated by this exercise:

Earth body, breathe breathe
body breath, the bird calls
seaweed unwinds, water flows
air brushes earth body
breathe gentle soft eternal light
beyond to the west
touch the unknown
touch gentle soft eternal light
beyond to the west, the west where life goes

Upon gentle waves sunlight dances
in its warmth the dolphin splashes
jumping over, then gliding into, the water

CLOSURE

When finishing up this session, suggest that each person refer to her drawing and her poem during the week to serve as a reminder to relax in a deep way. Close with a check-out circle, and if anyone needs special attention, place them in the center. Each person in the circle focus in your mind's eye on your drawing and recall your feelings of peace. Send that message to the person in the center. Do a movement together which is appropriate for making a transition into the outside world.

S U M M A R Y

The deep relaxation provided by the towelling exercise is the central focus of this class. In this session, each participant is given the opportunity to sense her own body and have her own experience. Do this massage-like exercise with a towel rather than with a direct hands-on approach to give participants an opportunity to experience movement free from the compulsion to respond to another person. The deep state of relaxation provided by the towelling gives rise to dances of physical, emotional, and mental release, which can enable us to experience pure awareness and peace. A unique aspect of this exercise is being able to engage one's consciousness in witnessing movement in its pure and natural state without any interference from the habituated mind. Finish the class with an expressive dance following the towelling exercise, a drawing, and a check-out regarding what happened during the class session.

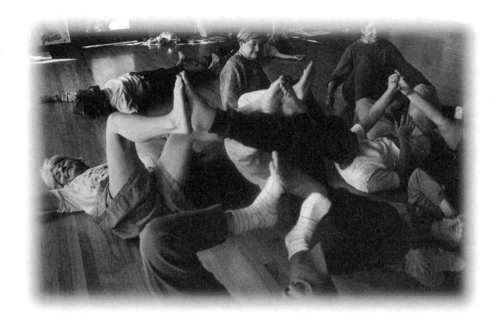

PLAYFUL INTIMACY AND HARMONIOUS INTEGRATION.

I was greatly elated by the discovery that there is a physiological basis for the ancient theory that laughter is good medicine."

— N O R M A N   C O U S I N S *from Anatomy of an Illness*

This is the final class in the series. The intention is to explore fun, humor, spontaneity, and play as a significant element in healing. I often ask people what they want to do in this particular class. One class said: laugh, dance, play, and not take ourselves so seriously. I tried to create a class that would do just that, and learned that closure through laughter and play is an excellent choice. This reminds people that their lives do not have to be all suffering and depression; that as long as there is life, there is also play, and laughter. It is also the intention of this class to create closure for the entire series, so we repeat the self-portrait exercise from the first class, and do a visualization that recalls all the places we have been since the class began.

C H E C K - I N

Do a special check-in for this final session: ask each person in the circle to do a spontaneous movement expressing how they feel right now. Add sounds and/or words as well. Everyone echo each other's movement until they have created a spontaneous group dance.

S E N S O R Y   A W A R E N E S S

1. Begin pulsing movements. Leader models this dance. Use sound.

2. Improvise on the pulse, using different parts of your body.

3. Shift into a shaking movement. Shake your hands, your arms, your shoulders, and your spine until your whole body is shaking.

4. Respond with whatever other movements arise from this shaking and pulsing.

If there is anyone in the class who is physically limited ask them to follow the movements while sitting in a chair.

M O V E M E N T   R E S O U R C E S

1. Walk and swing your arms. Walk any way you want.

2. Find another person to walk with and let one another's walk influence you.

3. Break contact and walk alone. Then find another person to walk with and develop your own movement together.

4. Repeat this until everyone has walked and moved together in partners.

5. Everyone hold hands and form a big open circle.

6. Rest. Look around and make eye contact with everyone. See and be seen.

7. Use a slower tempo and choose one person to lead the group in a simple movement that everyone else can follow in a conga line.

8. Whenever that person wants, go to the end of the line, and another person leads.

9. Repeat this until everyone has had a chance to be the leader.

There is another dance game called Stop, Look, and Listen. Here is how it works:

1. Everyone moves around freely until someone in the group calls out Stop, Look, Listen.

2. Everyone follows the direction.

3. The person who called out Stop! gives a direction and tells everyone what to do, i.e., everyone roll on the floor, everyone pretend that you are a monkey...

4. The group continues to do the movement until someone else calls out Stop, Look, Listen.

5. This goes on and on until finally a direction is called that everyone likes so much that they continue to do it without stopping.

This can be a very funny expression of the group mood. Here's another possible dance game. It's called Soul Train, and it's a great way for people to be outrageous and playful. The group forms two lines with an open corridor between them. Two people at one end of each line come dancing and prancing down the middle, improvising their movements. It is often done by using exaggerated attitudes such as silly, haughty, cool, sexy, tough, mean, and so forth. If the group is ready, sometimes no structure at all will be required. Just turn on some wonderful fun music and the group will know exactly what to do.

After this energetic dancing, take a break.

M O V E M E N T   M E D I T A T I O N

1. Find a comfortable place and lie down.

2. Focus on your feet. Where are they? What shape and color are they?

3. Move your feet around. Pay attention to how your foot connects to your lower legs, and your lower legs connect to your knees and your thighs.

4. Bring your attention to your legs. How do they feel? Move them around to get a better sense of them. How big or tall or wide or small is your leg? What is its shape?

5. Bring your attention to your pelvis. Sense how your leg connects to your pelvis. Move your pelvis. As it moves, pay attention to the connection between your pelvis and your legs, and your pelvis and your spine.

6. Bring your awareness to your breath. Bring your breath into your spine and your ribcage and up into your shoulders. Then bring your breath from your shoulders to your arms, and out into your fingers. Sense yourself in the joints of your arms.

Take your time, and allow people to absorb your suggestions. Give them time to record your words in their own inner voice. Speak softly enough that your comments register as suggestions, but not so softly that they have to strain to hear you.

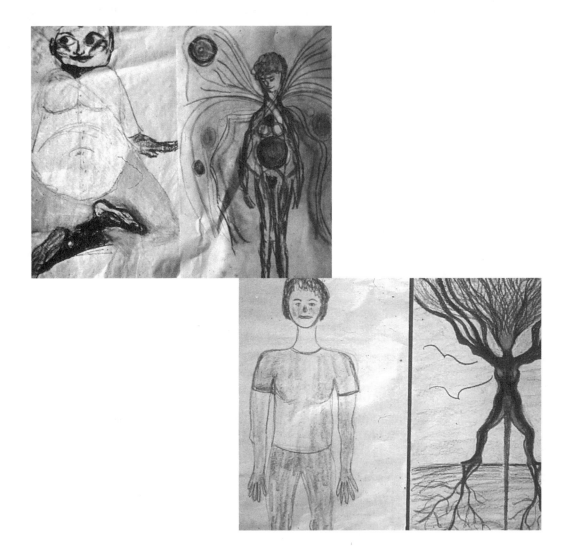

Amazing change can happen in just 5 days.
These are two before and after Self-Portraits.

G U I D E D   I M A G E R Y

The next part of the movement meditation is a guided image. Participants are still lying on their backs and can shift to another position. Before you begin this part of the exercise, which involves the imagination and creativity, awaken the sensations in their bodies. Although I am writing down different steps you might take to guide them, it is very important that here you use your own creativity. Create an exercise that applies to the series you have been teaching, and use this text as an example of how to do this. This is a review summary. Take relaxed time between each suggestion.

1. Take a moment to call forth your special animal ally. Call it by name and ask it to come and visit you again just so you know that it's there.

2. Remember your prayer. Take a moment to honor the spirit of your life force.

3. See yourself in your sacred place in nature.

4. Let your body relax, and with your observing mind, witness your breath.

5. Breathe in through your nose.

6. Pause.

7. Breathe out through your mouth.

8. Empty your breath, and linger in the emptiness.

9. As your breath returns, follow its movement and fill your whole being with breath.

10. With your eyes closed, look at yourself from the inside. Feel yourself from the inside. Imagine yourself from the inside.

11. Look at yourself from the outside. What do you look like? What do you feel like ?

12. Where are you? What is your environment?

SECOND SELF-PORTRAIT

Have paper and crayons out and ready. You might want to use a larger piece of paper than usual, or have masking tape available in case someone wants to tape two pieces together and draw on a bigger canvas. The next part of the exercise is to draw a second self-portrait. This gives a great insight into the participant's development during the weeks of the series.

1. When you are done with the visualization, open your eyes and begin to draw a second self-portrait. The first self-portrait was done at the beginning of the series. You will have thirty minutes to complete it.

2. When you are finished, look at your drawing and write down single words. Out of these single words, write a story, poem, chant, song.

3. Work in partners, sharing your drawings and dancing them. Give yourselves the necessary amount of time to do this exercise fully.

4. Share your self-portrait drawing with the group.

5. If the group is small, have each person dance her self-portrait for the whole group.

Here are some of the things people found in dancing and drawing on this final day: One woman drew rainbow wings, which for her were an image of hope, optimism, freedom, and independence. She drew a shackle on her leg but the chain was broken. Another woman drew solid feet in her self-portrait; she felt a connection to the earth. In her first self-portrait, she had drawn herself without any feet. Her head was drawn symmetrically and erect for the first time. Someone who had drawn only a face in her first self-portrait now drew a whole body. In every case, the images were more alive, fuller, more colorful, and expressive of a bigger-than-life picture of themselves than in the one at the beginning of the series.

1. Come into a circle once again to acknowledge yourselves and one another.

2. Do a slow movement, starting with your arms at your sides and pointing towards the earth. Slowly raise your arms to bring up energy from the earth and each other in the group. Place your hands together overhead and draw the energy from above,

like water cascading over your head and sweeping lightly over your face and body.

3. Breathe into your hands, press them into your hearts and share a moment of silence, then throw the arms into the air with a soft PAH! sound originating in your breath. Give a symbolic meaning to the "PAH!" sound, such as sending a message to a loved one, connecting to a higher life-force, or something meaningful to your group.

S U M M A R Y

On this final day of class, participants have a moment of celebration and levity with one another. In the opening moments of class, play movement games, or allow for open movement. Awaken the senses and dance a celebratory dance with one another. Lead participants into the second self-portrait through a guided meditation that helps them recall the material from previous sessions: animal ally, prayer, deep relaxation, the immune system, dances with nature, and the body as healer. This final class should pull in elements from all the previous classes, which will help the participant remember where they have been and what they are taking with them. This is also a time when you can more overtly model specific behaviors that function as metaphors for the participants: joining the celebration dance with them rather than being a passive onlooker gives participants an idea that they can collaborate on their healing process with their doctors and care-givers.

THE NEXT STEP IN HEALING

Dance Rituals for Community

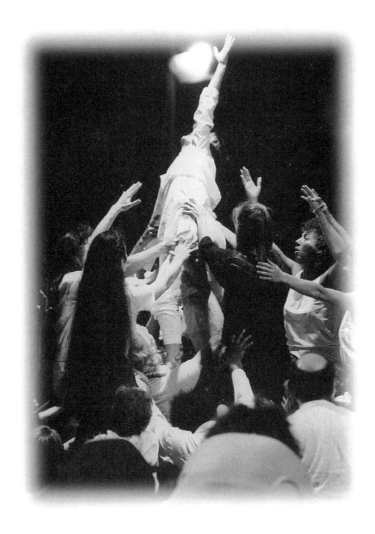

COMMUNITY PARTICIPATION

LINKS COMMON HUMANITY.

The community takes care

The community takes care of itself

A healthy community takes care

A healthy community takes care of itself

And when there is danger, when there is danger present,

A healthy community takes care of itself.

— A L L A N   S T I N S O N

from Circle the Earth, Dancing with Life on the Line

I imagine that when more of us begin to understand dance as a healing art, there will be a natural growth toward dance as a community art. This will be the next step in the evolution of reclaiming dance as a useful part of our lives. First, we must learn how dance can help us heal our bodies and our psyches; then, I believe, we will come to see how dance can be an active and creative force in the healing of our communities. I have made a number of experiments in this arena, which I want to share with you. They are related to the work documented in this book with people with life-threatening illness because they approach dance in the same way: as a vehicle for transformation and healing.

What I have learned from working with people who are facing their mortality is that an enormous isolation and fear must be faced, both by the people who are ill, and by those who care for them. During a dance workshop, a caregiver once confessed angrily that she did not like to be around people who were ill because it made her depressed and angry. Then she looked at her terminally ill dance partner, tears filling her eyes, and said, "I'm afraid to get too close to you because when you die, the pain will be more then I can bear." Speaking this truth is often painful. Relationships with friends and family change when you have cancer. In this culture, isolation is often intrinsic to the pain of the illness itself. This isolation is what we have to combat. Once I recognized this, I began to dream of the possibility of extending healing to include not only support groups for people with cancer or AIDS, but events in which the larger numbers of people whose lives were affected by these illnesses could also be healed.

I began to see how healing must take place and be integrated not only within our individual selves, but also within our communities, and in relation to the environments in which we live. We are by nature tribal creatures, and we are essentially part of the land on which we live. I do not believe it is healthy for us to live isolated or alone, in family units separate from our neighbors or disconnected from our environment. Yet, in our urban and suburban society, most of us have become fragmented, indifferent, alienated from each other, and lacking any sense of healthy community. We end up frustrated and powerless to control the fate of our lives and our environment. Through my desire to combat these realities, my work grew to explore the possibilities of community rituals and dances.

In 1976 and again in 1977, I and a collective of artists designed a day-long Citydance that took place throughout the various neighborhoods of San Francisco. In preparation for this event, a series of public workshops were offered at the San Francisco Museum of Modern Art to build a common language through movement and to develop a sense of how we could dance together as a community. Attendance ranged from 100 to 500 people, and out of the workshop grew the Citydance performance. On the day of the Citydance, I and my collaborators walked around the city like the Pied Pipers of Hamlin, drawing in people all along the way. The dance culminated in a triumphant celebration in a large plaza of downtown San Francisco. Citydance took place at the time of the murders of Mayor George Moscone and Supervisor Harvey Milk. The dance was intended to heal our wounds, and bring about peace and trust between people after these shocking and traumatic events.

The feelings generated by this large community using dance as a medium of transformation were extraordinary. The energy level was beyond anything I had imagined. I learned that there is a singular power in large groups of people with a common intention. I knew I wanted to learn to use that power to heal. What I learned through the Citydance process about community creation laid the foundation for other community-based dance rituals I have done. Over the next ten years, I made many other dance experiments with large groups. The most evolved one is called Circle the Earth, which began as a dance to reclaim a mountain in my community from the grips of a stalking killer. Out of that piece and my dream of using dance as a community healing, came a dance ritual called Dancing With Life on the Line. This dance was performed first in

1989, and again in 1991, and it grew out of many years of working with people with cancer and AIDS. I wanted to make a dance that would acknowledge these tragedies, and bring people together as a community for healing our separateness.

What I learned about community dances had taught me that when many people participate in the dance in order to actually bring about change in the lives of the participants and its witnesses, a critical mass of people will generate an extraordinary amount of power. To attract a larger community of participants, a public notice went out with the following message: "For many years, Circle the Earth has been danced for the well-being of the planet. Within this circle of health, peace and trust which we want to embody, there has emerged a parallel circle of death and isolation, ignorance and fear. To survive this crisis, the first circle must be strengthened: the second circle, broken. We ask you to dance with those among us who are fighting for our lives, to support this commitment and honor the courage of those living with cancer and HIV/AIDS. We all have war, doubt, struggles and pain. Only by crossing the lines that we draw between us, only by joining together in action, in feeling and with spirit can there ever be an end to any of it." 135 people responded! 135 people danced, and 1,000 people came to support and witness their performance. Many kinds of people came to dance: people with cancer and other life-threatening illness; people with AIDS and their caregivers and friends; people ranging from age 14 to age 75; men and women of all backgrounds; dancers and non-dancers.

The impact was tremendous. One participant said, "My life has been changed! I feel that I have a sense of purpose which I had completely lost. The support of the community gave this to me." Another participant wrote in her journal, "In community, we can share all our resources to meet all our needs. Through community, our connection with all of life is made manifest." One young man with AIDS had a T-cell count of 40 at the beginning of the preparatory workshop. After the performance, his T-cell count went up to 240! The community that gathered together created such a positive force that people in the dance stayed together in different sub-groups and continued to meet and dance and do ritual together throughout the year.

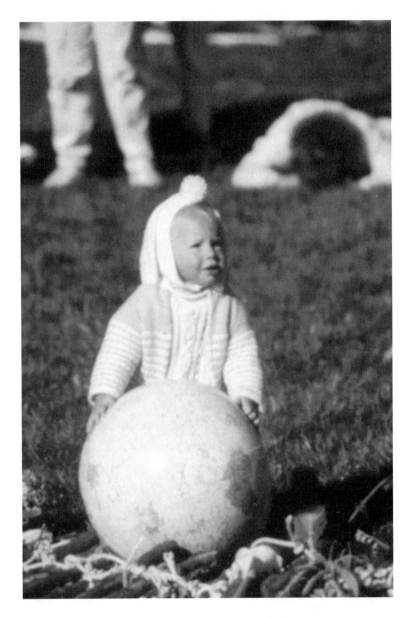

There is a special dance for children—our hope for the future.

GLOBAL HEALING

This community dance sparked many, many more. One particular dance that is related to Circle the Earth is called the Planetary Dance. As Circle the Earth began to spread, and people from around the world wanted to find a way to participate, I excerpted one of the dances from Circle the Earth and suggested that people replicate this form in their communities, imbuing it with symbols and meanings that pertained to their environment, their community, and their lives. This idea spread like wildfire, and now every year, the Planetary Dance, done every spring to invoke the spirits of the earth and ourselves in a ritual of healing, renewal of community, and affirmation of life, is performed around the world in 36 different countries. When we dance the Planetary Dance at our chosen site, each participant dances for someone or something they deeply care about. Some people dance for loved ones who have died during the past year; others dance for the healing of the environment, or for the health of people with AIDS and cancer. There is a special dance for the children, who might dedicate their dance to the wildflowers, to their pets, to a world without smoking, to the dolphins. Everyone chooses a dedication to something bigger than themselves; the dance becomes a prayer.

And so the healing circle grows.

I encourage you to take your desire for change and healing as far as you dare. Everything you have learned and everything you know applies to this much-needed art form. Your experiments bring us closer to a new understanding of dance as a healing art, the power of community, and the will of the people as a positive agent for change.

> *The spirit of the well is deep. The well of the spirit is deeper still.*
> *May the spirit that brought us together, keep us together*
> *And keep us well all along the way*
>
> — ALLAN STINSON, *from Circle the Earth*

REUNITING DANCE AND MEDICINE

My Conversation with a Bear Dancer Physician

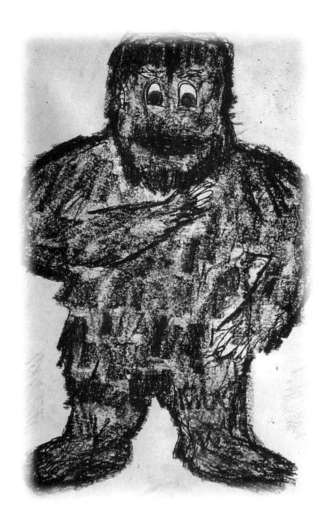

"MY BEAR IS FRIGHTENING AND BIGGER THAN LIFE AND FIERCE. BUT IT IS
ONLY HIS APPEARANCE THAT IS SCARY. ON THE INSIDE HE IS SOFT AND LOVING.
HE CAN TAKE CARE OF ME AND SEE THAT NO HARM COMES TO ME."
A PARTICIPANT FINDS AN ANIMAL ALLY.

One of my colleagues and supporters in this work has been Dr. Mike Samuels. I feel it is important to include a short excerpt of his essay so we can hear from another voice, a voice that speaks from his experience as a physician. Dr. Samuels has discovered art and ritual as a powerful tool for healing. Recently, we had an opportunity to share our ideas on this subject. In the course of our conversation we talked of our dilemma and frustraton over terminology. If we use the word art, many readers would make the assumption that we meant only the visual arts. However, both of us use art to include dance, music, poetry, story telling, architecture, and environment. This combination I refer to as the expressive arts. Who do we mean when we talk of the artist? The artist could be a trained professional dancer, painter, musician, poet, story teller, etc. But just as true, the artist is in all of us. We are all artists. It is our birth right.

Ritual is another word that needs a new definition. The dictionary places its emphasis on the more traditional religious rites and this can be misleading. Ritual, as I use the term, refers to an artistic process by which people gather and unify themselves in order to confront the challenges of their existence. In this definition, ritual dance can be a transformative force in healing. Art is an idiosyncratic form, but unlike ritual, healing is not always its primary intention. Dr. Samuels elaborates on these thoughts. I find his own theory of the bridge between art and science of particular interest for us as teachers in this field. In a culture that places such importance on the scientific world, the biological and physiological insights on the creative and artistic process can fortify our belief in our work.

Mike and I have been friends for a long time and I thought I knew him and his work very well. I was wrong. I had no idea that Mike was a bear dancer. The story of the bear dance unfolded during one of our conversations. I was telling him that although the complementary therapies are slowly being acknowledged by the medical profession, the full impact of dance as a healing force is still held in the dark. At this point he began to tell me the story of his bear dance. Having identified the bear as his animal ally in this work (see chapter 11, "Finding Your Animal Ally," for further reference to this topic), he was looking for a bear skin to use as a costume to wear whenever he performed his bear dance. I thought to myself, where would anyone find something as unusual as a bear skin? Well, he had heard of an Indian trader in New Jersey and traveled there to see him. He told the trader his story and his interest in dancing and ritual as healing. The trader was so impressed that he went into his back room and came out with a magnificent bear skin which he gave to him as a gift. Now he wears it whenever he does this dance. He particularly enjoys doing his bear dance at the children's ward in hospitals and encourages the children to wear the bear skin and do the dance themselves. Some of the ideas we talked about during our informal conversation are being presented here as an introduction to his essay.

MIKE: All of us are trying to figure out a way to free the inner healer to produce those toxins that kill the cancer and dance is the most efficient way we now have.

ANNA: You really believe that?

MIKE: Yeah, I really think that. That's why I'm doing this work.

ANNA: That is amazing. A dancing doctor.

MIKE: Ritual...see dance to me is part of ritual.

ANNA: Yes, that is exactly how I work with dance. Dance is an integration of all the arts and consequently of the whole person. That is where its power to heal lies.

MIKE: That's right. Dance is the kinesthetic body part of ritual. A ritual is whole; it's higher in a world experience. It becomes very real through its costume, its movement, its sights, its smells, its belief system, its story, its poetry, its song, and every single thing you do within it. They all add to its reality until it becomes so real that it actually becomes reality itself. When it becomes reality itself, body physiology thinks it's reality and responds by changing. Dance does it best of all forms because body movement probably has the most brain power associated with it. In imagery studies, the image is very dim in the "imagery state." An actual muscle movement in dance, on the other hand, is not dim at all—it's a big amount of neural input. That's why it's more effective than pure imagery by itself.

ANNA: Yes. When you dance the image, you embody it totally. The physical dimension releases emotional responses that really bring the image to life.

MIKE: I think that the whole thing we are trying to do is to be one with something. You want to be absolutely one with that state without a rational mind interfering, without a separation, in old Zen-Buddhist terms or something. You want a complete belief system to occur. Dance is a terrific way to do that.

In the following essay excerpt, Dr. Samuels discusses his ideas. His writing has been included here not only as an important resource for us as teachers, but also with the hope that through "spreading the word," in the future, other doctors may be encouraged to "dance in his footsteps."

DANCE AS A HEALING FORCE

An Essay by Mike Samuels, M.D.

When I refer to "art" in this essay I mean all the arts:
dance, music, painting, sculpture, storytelling, poetry, architecture,
and environment. All of these forms are art.

Art, prayer, and healing; all come from the same source—the human soul. The energy that fuels these processes is the basic force of life, of creativity, of love. Deep within us we have memory of a beautiful place where our spirits were given breath. We are connected to the soul of God in the deepest marrow of our being. By traveling inside ourselves, we can glimpse the deep spaces of our lives, feel them, live in them. We can bring back their memory and their spirit, through art and ritual.

I believe that the voices of the inner world speak to us in a language most similar to art. It is below words, above silence, and close to poetry. It is God singing and dancing. It is our soul listening. It is the voice of the life force, of expansion and love within us. When we pray, when we travel inward and heal, we can bring back traces of pure spirit. Art and ritual are the voices of the spirit. They are the energy of healing. Art and healing are lovers, tied together with a silver thread, and bound irreversibly through time. Today the artist and the healer are feeling the rebirth of this ancient connection. In an age where art has become decorative and lost its spiritual meaning, in an age where medicine has lost its connection to the heart and the intuitive spirit, art and healing can be reunited through ritual to become one again.

If the force is love, and the voice is the soul, its language art and ritual, and its product healing, where are we going? How is ritual coming into the medical center, or healing coming into the artist's studio? Art and ritual are the doorways into the realm of the heart, the tool for transformation we now seek. They are what opens and what changes. When a patient in a cancer ward is visited by an artist, lets herself move into the land of spirit, then lets a piece of art come out into the world and cries and is touched for the first time since she has been in the hospital, a healing has taken place. She has opened her heart to love. Ritual as the vehicle through which an open heart can enter medicine is very real. In love we need a lover and a loved one; in healing we need a healer and a person who needs healing. Here, the bridge is art and ritual, the language of love. How do art and ritual heal? How can an image change reality? How does experiencing an image or moving through a dance ritual actually change our body's physiology? We are just beginning to understand the answers to these questions. Let me describe how the body physically and physiologically deals with the phenomenon of imagery and movement.

Thoughts, emotions, and images form in different areas of the brain and involve different neurotransmitters. Images of movement and dance are held in areas of the brain responsible for instigating muscle movement. A discharge of neurons comes from both an instigation of movement and its memory. This is experienced by the person as an image of movement coming from her imagination or her memory. Since dance involves so many proprioceptive sensory and motor pathways, both imagining and remembering a movement is very real and intense when experienced. The movements are reflected as discharges in areas of the brain that send messages to muscles. Even though the dancer does not move, the proper muscles will respond microscopically. The place where the images of movement are held send nerve messages to the hypothalamus which go out to the rest of the body. Likewise, the movement itself is picked up by the brain and sends messages to the hypothalamus. A dancer sends out messages to her whole body when she moves or remembers a movement. In the areas of the brain that control movement and the memory of movement, nerve cells discharge and images come to life.

The hypothalamus activates the autonomic nervous systems resulting in the arousal or realization of a "double balancing" system which reaches out to the whole body, touching virtually every cell. The sympathetic branch is the branch of the fight or flight reaction. An image in the big brain of a threat alerts the hypothalamus to cause sympathetic arousal. This speeds up the heartbeat, increases breathing, sends blood to the large muscles, floods the body with adrenaline and hormones, and creates a state of alertness. The memory of moving away from a threat, or facing it and fighting, releases tension and puts the person in a state of release. The stimulation of the parasympathetic nervous system results in relaxation, healing, and maintenance. Heartbeat and blood pressure slows, breathing slows, blood goes to the intestines.

This oversimplified model gives an idea of how the mind is connected to the body, and how muscle movements stimulate the whole body. When a person dances or imagines dancing, the area of the cerebrum that holds images of muscle movement is stimulated and sends messages to the hypothalamus. This allows us to respond to the dance imagery. If the dance image is one of deep joy or release, the body is put in a healing state through the hypothalamic pathways. If it is one of persistent fear or tension, the body remains tense and in the physiology of stress. In addition, the body can bathe every cell in the body with a hormonal flood as the imagery of threat or love lights up the neural nets in the brain. As this flashes through us, the hypothalamus sends messages to the adrenal glands to release epinephrine, adrenaline, and other hormones which go throughout the body and are picked up by receptors in our cells, causing some cells to contract, others to relax, some to act, others to rest. Our entire physiology is changed a second time by an image or dance movement held in our consciousness, and to it we respond.

Another realm is that of the neurotransmitter. Images cause specific areas of the brain itself to release endorphins and other neurotransmitters which affect brain cells and the immune system. The neurotransmitters relieve pain and make the immune system function more efficiently. They make killer cells eat cancer cells, white blood cells attack the HIV virus, and generally change the body's ability to respond to illness. When a person dances, or imagines a dance movement which is freeing or which brings out inner healing images, the body actually changes its physiology in response. A person need not do anything, the body will do it just through the impetus of dancing or imagining movement.

How does healing occur? The resonating body/mind/spirit balances our physiology by the threefold path we mentioned above: thoughts in the brain; autonomic nervous system balance, hormonal balance and neurotransmitter balance; cellular change. What are images and how do they relate to healing? I divide imagery into two basic types—receptive and programmed. Receptive imagery comes to you, bidden or unbidden, and rests in your mind's eye. It can come onto a blank screen and appear as itself, or it can come over your thoughts and appear mixed. Programmed imagery is different. You choose an image and hold it in your thoughts for a reason. The choice may be deliberate or you may choose an image that comes to you from a receptive place. Either way, the image affects your world. How does this happen? The image affects your body by the threefold path. Images affect your world by giving you ideas to plan from, emotional motivation to continue, and meaning. When a person gets an image of the future, then she can make it happen. Magic is the image becoming real in the outer world.

Healers work with imagery by having a patient picture her illness, her healing forces, and the healing process in their mind's eye. First, the patient imagines what the illness looks like in as much detail as they can. Next, they imagine how the body's resources could deal with the visualized illness. This is done as a process over time. Biologically based imagery is effective when it is anatomically accurate and detailed. Researchers have found that when imagery is very specific, picturing, for example, one type of white blood cell, it alone is found to change. Next, patients are encouraged to allow metaphorical imagery to form. This is the state where little men, dogs, or white light blast, eat, or dissolve blackness, mud, or other little men. This metaphorical imagery often takes place spontaneously after the biological imagery. Finally, patients can hold a programmed image in mind. They can picture themselves healed, surrounded by white light, as God, as a power animal, or being strong and secure.

Healing art can be used by a patient in two obvious ways. The images can be viewed and allowed to change a person's consciousness, or images can be used to help a person visualize the healing process or a healed state. Imagery is healing if it puts a person in an altered state, relaxes them, opens their heart, or gives them energy. Monet's Water Lilies was so relaxing that patients would visit them in museums and sit and meditate in front of them for hours. The third way art heals a viewer is by showing a patient images that move them. When patients with breast cancer see art, music, or dance made by breast cancer patients, it opens them up to emotions they may have hidden. This allows them to discuss these emotions with their families, support people, and healers. Patients who have a particular illness are moved by art that portrays other people's experiences with the same illness. It makes them feel connected, relieves isolation, and releases deep emotions. This type of art can be very disturbing for other people to view. This imagery is not for relaxation or transcendence; it is for opening the heart.

All of these kinds of art work by changing consciousness, freeing energy, and awakening the spirit to resonate with the body/mind. They are technologies for using ritual as healing. Imagery can be most powerful when it comes from the inner world of the person who is ill. It is direct, meaningful, and sometimes more effective than other images. However, images made by artists can be so powerful, that they can transform, even though they are not personal to the patient.

Throughout recorded history, artists have believed that their images have power in themselves. The shaman was the first artist and healer. The shaman traveled inward, glimpsed the spirits, acted, brought back the healing, and made art. He or she told the tale, crafted the masks, danced the song, and brought the inner world outward through ritual. Shamanic ritual was believed to actually have the power to change the physical world. What is going on now that has caused the growth of ritual and healing worldwide? Why are you reading this book and doing dance ritual as a healing art? Art and ritual as a healing force is being born as we speak. The concept is catching fire, awakening people's spirits. The idea is being born in the world of the artist, and the world of the healer. Art in the hospital, or art at the bedside of a person who is ill, is an electrifying experience. It becomes a doorway to the spirit, a vehicle for the opening of the heart. It is integral to healing. There are now artists making healing art purposely. It is a whole new field in art. This work, as I see it, heals the artist, or the world. It works by freeing the artist's own healing energy, and resonating with their body, mind, and spirit. The artist can also make art to heal another person, or a group of people. This is a transpersonal healing, the art of interconnection which joins us at our centers. Thus art heals by releasing the energy of the viewer, relaxing her, allowing something within her to be freed, resonating with their body, mind, and spirit. Another type of art heals the world, like the Planetary Dance referred to in the chapter "The Next Step in Healing." The artist works with the energy of the whole system, whether it be a neighborhood, an ecosystem, or the planet itself. This art can be ceremonial, environmental, performative, or static. It involves the community, energy, and movement. It is truly shamanic; it balances the world.

The second category of healing art is the art patients create to heal themselves. Art at the bedside, dance with cancer patients, art workshops, art and dance therapy, exhibitions at hospitals, and environments created in healing centers, all represent this type. It does not matter whether healing art is made by an artist or a patient. The cancer patient who dances frees her inner artist and her inner healer; the ancient movements allow her to change, physiologically, and spiritually. This is not a passive art form. Healing art is not meant to be watched. It is the life force. This art is made to change reality. It has the power to transform.

We are on the doorstep of a great journey. Anna Halprin's work is one of its first steps. Imagine where we can go from here. Imagine art, music, and dance in every hospital, art for anyone who is ill. Imagine lifting the spirits of someone who is about to die. Imagine being in love.

MIKE SAMUELS, M.D.
*Director, **Art as a Healing Force**, California*

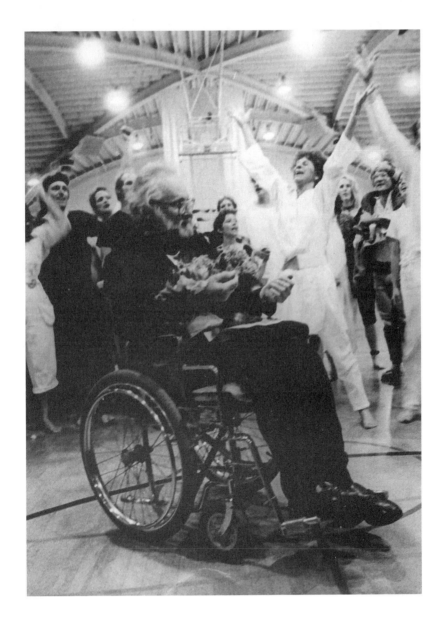

No-one an outsider.

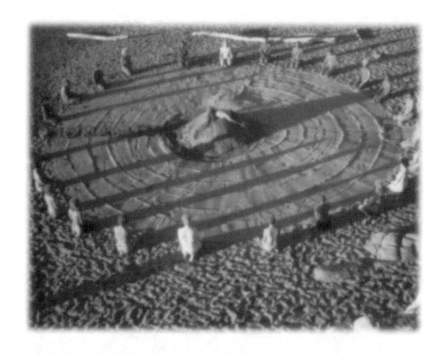

A   G R O U P   R I T U A L .

"In healing, everything is possible, even as nothing is certain."

— MAUREEN REDL

One of the challenges of working with people with life-threatening illness is the frequent distance between the content of my class plans, and what I am actually greeted with when I walk into a classroom. Sometimes this gap is frighteningly large. There have been times when I have come to class, and all the lesson plans in the world won't help me with the reality of the situation I have to face. Someone has died; someone is dying; someone is filled with dread about dying. This is part of what it means to work with people with life-threatening illness; we always have to face death and our fear of it as we continue to live.

The lessons detailed in the earlier chapters of this book are important, but they aren't the whole story when working with people with life-threatening illness. It is crucial to respond with as much alertness and compassion as possible to the issues of life and death that emerge while doing this work. I try to bring all of my experiences and resources as a teacher, artist, cancer survivor, and human being into the classroom with me. My practice is to become as sensitive as I can to the fear of death, which is expressed at some point by everyone challenging a life-threatening illness.

People ask me if one has to be a cancer survivor to do this kind of work. I don't think you do, but I know that you must be willing to confront your own attitudes around death, and face your own issues surrounding some of life's most revealing questions. You will surely be deeply touched by the stories, the dances, and the participants. I know that I have been. And I have learned that we must allow ourselves to experience the intensity of our own feelings; not to distance ourselves with an attitude of pity, but rather to legitimately feel fear, sadness, or joy as these feelings touch places in our own lives. Many issues will come up for you. It is very important to keep growing and experiencing this process of yourself. Dance, move, draw, and write to keep yourself evolving. Doing this work will also help you keep burn-out at bay. The process is nourishing, and will give back to you some of what you give to your students.

When I first began to work with people with life-threatening illness, I felt very responsible. I thought that this kind of teaching required a depth and perfection that called upon a great deal of planning, preparation, clarity, and "doing the right thing." In the beginning, planning my lessons in advance and working within these known parameters gave me a sense of security. As I gained some experience, I began to trust my more spontaneous responses to the people with whom I worked. It is still important for me to plan my classes and to be aware of the specific issues pertaining to people with life-threatening illness, but my ability to be spontaneous adds to my teaching in a positive way.

I have discovered certain principles useful in teaching expressive movement upon which I constantly rely. They include:

- *Returning to my body* as a way to respond to the moment. How has this story or situation affected me? How do I feel, and what can I do for myself that will respond to the moment? What are my personal resources? Will my personal responses work for the group?

- *Empathy.* Listen intently to the words each person has chosen. Listen to the tone of voice, and watch the body language and the reaction of the group. Engage in this person's experience from the inside.

- *Find a container.* My contribution as a teacher is to offer a container in the form of an activity that will allow each person and the group as a whole to express themselves, and release and transform their stuck places or self-destructive forces. The container is comprised of the expressive arts media—movement, drawing, writing, sounding (singing, chanting), storytelling, speaking. No two people are alike. It is important to recognize that each person lives in her own unique body with her own individual responses. You can instruct people in what to do without telling them how to do it. This openness will enable your participants to tap into their own meaningful imagery, feelings, and movement. For example, a direction like "rise and let go," tells participants what to do. One person may do the movement while sitting, another might stand, another may move through space. Some might join others, others choose to remain alone.

- *Trust the process.* When in doubt, move, draw, write, speak. Remember that you don't have to control or manipulate the process, and that you are not expected to know all the answers ahead of time. You are facilitating a process unfolding in front of you. Trust that the process of dancing, writing, drawing, and speaking will yield the healing that is needed.

I always return to these parameters; I constantly recombine them in new ways, depending upon the situation I encounter. This open-ended way of teaching enables me to respond specifically to what is happening in the room. My approach has become more open-ended and my flexibility serves my students as well.

There is a fine balance between responding to the moment and working with the themes I have established as core to the experience of life-threatening illness. Flexibility does not eliminate the need for the kinds of planning the earlier parts of this book present, but it does make it possible to respond more sincerely to people's responses and feelings as they arise. The single most important thing you can do as a teacher in this situation is to respond to the moment as it unfolds, using all of your resources to facilitate its transformation.

The following four stories describe actual teaching situations I have encountered, and how I adapted my pre-conceived lesson plans to respond to the needs of the participants. As you will see, they all involve a creative response to the revelation of people's fear about death, transformation, and dying. They have been written in such a way to give you insight not only into what I did, but why I did it, a living laboratory of theory into practice. The ordinary type describes what actually happened in the class; the writing in italics represents my inner process, and how I came to make my decisions about the classroom activities. My hope is that these examples will enable you to use your skills and imagination, and gain the confidence necessary to create your own responses.

A DEATH IN THE GROUP

Peggy Rogers, Director of Client Services at the Menlo Park Cancer Support and Education Center, came to me before class one day to let me know that someone in the group had died. She asked me if I had a ritual for this kind of a situation. This was the first time I had worked with this particular group. I didn't know them; they didn't know me; I didn't know the person who died. I don't have a formula for creating rituals to use on the spot. But this situation was presented to me, and this is what happened.

As the class began, people sat in chairs in the circle. In a very sensitive way, Peggy let people know what had happened. Everybody sat very quietly; the room was absolutely still. This was a group of people who had worked together for a long time. They were very close to one another; this was akin to a death in the family. On this somber note, I introduced myself briefly, said I didn't know the deceased person myself, but I imagined it was very sad for all of them to lose a member of their group.

I approached the situation as one of grief and loss, rather than one of death itself.

The first thing I asked them to do was to stand. I told them that standing is a way of honoring someone.

Standing conveys respect. In my own tradition, we honor the memory of someone who has passed by standing for certain prayers. We stand when we salute the flag. In the Native American tradition, people stand when different tribes enter the pow-wow. The group needed to take a special stance in response to this death. It wasn't appropriate that we remain sitting. I also imagined that standing might evoke a response from them; they seemed frozen by the news of this death. Standing can initiate movement. It is also a posture which implies rising up.

We stood in a circle, and held hands.

Circles are ways for people to gather in unity. I remember when I was in the hospital and my mother came to see me after my operation. I was in pain, and emotionally drained. The first thing I said to her when she walked into my room was, "Hold my hand." I know from experience that hand-holding is very comforting.

I encouraged the members of the group to bring the spirit and memory of Mary (not her real name) into the center of our circle as they inhaled deeply. I said "As you inhale, bring your memories of Mary into yourself. When you exhale, imagine that those memories are moving into our circle. All our memories are going to be gathered together."

I went to the breath to help people find release. Connecting to the breath is especially important because it relieves anxiety and offers nourishment. Breathing deeply relaxes tension, changes consciousness, and is an essential way to return to the body, the home of the self. Evoking memory helps the group to embrace memories of their friend. Sharing memories and gathering them in a circle creates a collective experience of appreciation, and loving feelings.

I asked if they would let out a sigh or a sound as they exhaled. This would be a way of sending our thoughts and voices to Mary. Sounding is a personal and collective opportunity to express, reinforce, and deepen the quality of feelings. There may be inhibition about making sounds; people are afraid of being heard. Adding music to this kind of exercise may help liberate people's voices. If people are unaccustomed to using their voices with movement, with a little coaxing, working with the voice and with the body can become a rich and emotional experience.

I heard the quality of the group's feelings in their chant. In response, I suggested a swaying movement.

Their chant was nostalgic. It wasn't sad. It wasn't mournful. It was sweet and gentle. I imagined Mary as a gentle person. The movement of swaying seemed to suit the energy of the song.

The group began to sway from side to side. I danced and moved with them, and then began to develop the movement, adding the arms and the head, getting bigger and varying the dynamics. The group began to follow.

I felt that they still needed me to direct them toward an expression of their feelings, so I began to dance too, modeling different possibilities of movement for them. I am always observing for the moment when I can step back and let them take over.

I asked them to move with the sounds they were making.

I knew that movement would help them continue to develop their song, and that the song would help them develop their movement.

The chant and movement built up. We found a strong beat in the dance as the dynamics became strong and people began moving with their feelings. Their strength went into their legs and feet, adding more zest to the body. I played music that supported their rhythmic expression.

Their mood was changing. Whenever you get the pulse going, it indicates more energy and activity in the group. A pulse can be very motivating, leading to developing new movements.

As we danced and chanted, I invited people to speak out loud any of their memories of Mary. They did so with the chant in the background. This went on for a long time, because there were so many people in the group. They began to respond to one another's memories.

Sharing what they remembered about Mary felt like an appropriate way for them to have some closure with her through the dance.

I asked them to visualize Mary. What were her physical characteristics? How did her voice sound, or the way she laughed, or the way she cried? If they were to draw an image or picture in her memory, what would it be?

I was preparing to create an image. I felt the group had completed their collective physical expression. They needed to get back to themselves again and create something in her memory that would bring closure.

I asked them to recall Mary in her finest hour, or a moment of her inner beauty. I asked them to see her healthy and vibrant and to imagine her in a place in nature. I asked them to see her singing in the center of our circle, and dancing with us, free and spontaneous. I asked them to make a drawing of their feelings for her.

I didn't ask them to draw Mary. I asked them to express their feelings for Mary in their drawing. This allowed them to get back to their own experience of Mary, and what her death evoked in each of them.

Everyone shared their drawings in the circle. As they did, I said, "Let this drawing be a way to say good-bye to Mary." Some people wrote poems or messages for her. Some people began to cry when they showed their drawings. I gave the group an opportunity to imagine where she may have gone, and what that experience might be like. Many of the drawings expressed how they saw her now, in death.

I was tremendously moved by their commitment to her, and their love and care for her. I knew that the particular story they were sharing had to do with life after death. They were talking about Mary's death, but they were also talking about the mystery of grief, loss, and death, which involved us all. I saw this in the poems and the things they were actually saying. I began to think ahead while they were talking. What are we going to do with these drawings? They began to talk about Mary's husband who had been a member of their support group, and their concern for him. I didn't want to tell them what to do with their drawings - I wanted to suggest that their drawings had meaning for others as well as for themselves.

I suggested that they give the drawings to her husband, or put the drawings up in the rooms at the center, or keep the drawings for themselves. Some people chose to hang the drawings in the center to share with everyone, and some went to visit Mary's husband, and gave their drawings to him. They wanted to give their drawings to others as a symbol of their love for Mary, and their wishes for her safe passage to the other side.

I now felt we needed to bring this to a closure. We needed to release her.

I used a traditional Buddhist gesture in which you bring your hands into a prayer position in front of your heart, take a deep inhalation, and then on your exhalation, release your hands up to the sky with the sound of PAH! We added to this gesture all the images we had created. We imagined them all gathered in our hands and into our hearts, and as we did this, we sent our images out of our circle, and to Mary, wherever she was.

T R A N S F O R M I N G D E S P A I R

I was leading a group of people who were obviously in despair. Their check-ins revealed a great deal of distress and grief. Jeff, a young man with AIDS and bone cancer, shared with us that he had lost all purpose in life. He couldn't ride his bicycle anymore, or work with the children he loved. Formerly, he taught young children at the YMCA, and had spent much of his free time dancing or doing sports. He wasn't able to do any of the things that had made his life meaningful. Someone else shared her discouragement. She'd been in remission when her tests reported that the cancer had cropped up again. One after another, people shared stories of discouragement, despair, and a sense of giving up.

I do a lot of observing. I observe body language. I notice how people are sitting, whether they're sitting back, forward, up, or down. I notice whether or not their facial expressions around their eyes, lips, and jaws are ones of tension, or relaxation, or if they're staring off into space. I notice if there are any gestures or movements in their hands or feet, whether they're crossing their legs or arms, whether or not they're holding their breath. What seemed evident in this group was that people were withdrawn. Some were slouched over and looking down. Others looked concerned for the people who revealed their pain during the check-in. I observed that, and at the same time I observed myself. I noticed I was taking short breaths and I was anxious. I kept wringing or holding my hands. I noticed that I kept wanting to pay attention to my gut feelings.

I asked the group to take a deep breath together, and to let out a sigh.

I imagined that there was fear in the group, and that along with fear, there was explosiveness. Dealing with fear takes the appropriate container. I didn't go in that direction because I didn't sense a readiness in myself. I didn't see the fear; I imagined it. No one was sitting forward. No one was clenching their teeth or tensing their jaws or making a fist out of their hands or nervously jiggling their legs. I didn't want to force or invent a response. Instead, I heard people ready to die, ready to just give up the fight. I turned to myself and to my body. What does my body want to do? Is it possible to get to the breath? Would they take it and go with it? If they didn't, I knew I could let it go and try something else.

I said, "Let's go into the resignation and see where it takes us." If that isn't clear, I could have asked: "Where does your movement want to go?" We exhaled with a sigh. We then chose to take a great inhalation, contrasting the release of our exhale with the fullness of our inhale. That was uplifting.

The moment I inhaled, I noticed other people doing it. It just seemed to click. Now I could continue in this vein.

We began to develop the inhalation by bringing in the movements of the hands and arms.

I ask myself: Are people with me? Are they with the movement? I try to give clear directions so they can follow them without looking at me, so they can stay with their own experience. When I develop a movement from the breath, I listen to my body's signs and signals as resources.

We kept developing this movement, gradually adding our spines and our heads. As we exhaled, we let the movement drop into our shoulders. Before long, the movement became circular, with our arms lifting up as if in prayer, and then dropping down, as if gathering strength from the earth.

I chose to work with their despair, since this is what was being expressed, verbally and physically. I made choices from the tangible, identifiable clues they offered. If I had followed my imagination, I would have been imposing myself on them, and the movement we were doing might not have been congruent with their feelings. I know that if people are willing to do a movement as we were doing it—the lifting, exhaling and dropping—it must match an emotional response. Otherwise, there would be no motivation to follow it.

There are choices to be made all along the way. This is challenging because not everybody is in the same place at the same time. Some people may need to stay in the physical realm a lot longer, some people may be ready to start developing the movement into images. This presents another choice point. I ask myself, "How are we going to further integrate these images into their lives and experience?"

When I want to accommodate the different needs of the participants in developing the material, I simply say, "Feel free to develop this gathering and lifting and falling movement in any way that comes to you." Then I can witness them begin to develop the movement in their own way.

The moment I see people adding their own signature to the movement, I know that they must be working with an image, even though they may not be conscious of it. Otherwise why would one person be rippling when another is shaking? I began to see people working with images, and other people began searching for images.

This is another place where choice comes up: Where should we go next? I could say, "If you have an image that you're working from, just let that image take you further into the development of the movement. Rise out of your chair, move through space, make the sound of your image." If some people prefer the rising up, and some prefer the downward pull, I would encourage both of these developments.

I allowed people to explore their movement a bit longer, and then I brought them back together into a circle. People began to call out their particular images. As they began to develop these images in movement, I told them to feel free to interact with anyone else in the group.

I suggested interaction because I felt they needed some outside stimuli to extend their explorations. People were staying in the same place with their movements. Some people began to withdraw again. It seemed that they had developed their images as far as they could, and they didn't have the resources to go any further. I thought the stimulation of other people would help them respond more deeply to themselves.

As a result of the interaction in the group, the movement kept growing, changing, building, and so did their feelings. I asked people to draw their images and share them. Jeff, who had been so discouraged in the beginning of the class, drew a heart with hands reaching out. A transformation had taken place. He said he knew what his purpose was: to give and receive love. He looked radiant.

By using the movements of the ribcage that were involved with the rising and falling of the hands and arms, Jeff was able to connect to feelings of love and tenderness. Working with the arms also brings up feelings of reaching toward others. Jeff's image of the big heart and his reaching arms were a visual interpretation of this physical experience.

At the end of class, the mood in the room was completely different than it had been in the beginning. Each person had found some measure of beauty and meaning in their lives. They were no longer in a state of despair with its limited options, but full of hope and new possibilities.

W H O ' S   N E X T ?

I was meeting with a familiar group in a hospital setting. The spirit of this group was embodied in a woman named Kathy, who had been attending since 1992. While working with our animal allies, she discovered a turtle. The turtle had a large shell with a mandala pattern which protected her and where she could snuggle when she needed comfort. In 1992, she had been told by her doctors that she wouldn't live more than a couple of weeks. Armed with her turtle's protection and her fierce will, she was alive for five years after that. This story takes place in 1997, as her dying process began to deepen.

On this particular day, we noticed that Kathy wasn't there when class started, but we didn't pay too much attention because everyone in the group was straggling in at odd times. I made a series of false starts. I would do a check-in, and then someone else would come in and tell their story. The energy in the room was very fragmented, and I didn't have much sense of what to do. Then Kathy arrived, in a wheelchair. She had been getting progressively more frail, but this was this first time we had seen her this way.

As she arrived, she was talking in a loud and somewhat incoherent voice. She joined the circle, and continued to talk as if no one else was in the room. She complained that her legs were hurting. One of the assistants went to her side and started massaging her legs. She thought that was very good. She started flailing her arms in the air. What were we going to do? This person was the flame-keeper of the group, and there she was, incoherent, babbling, not making any sense. And yet, what was happening to her was very powerful and clear.

Everybody started looking at me, wondering what we were going to do. We were seeing a person whose illness had taken control of her life. It was a frightening moment for the group.

I didn't have the foggiest notion of what to do. I had so many feelings. I felt that this was the beginning of the end for Kathy. I didn't know how I was going to reach her. There were other people there too, and they had stories that needed to be told. I was confused, fragmented, and sad. I said to myself, "I don't know what to do. I'm just going to sit with how this is affecting me. I am giving up my role as the teacher. I will just let everybody sit with this, as I am doing, until I feel I can move."

So we sat. This gave us all permission to do nothing except be there with her and be present. As she slowly shifted her awareness to the group, we went on. There were other people who had stories to tell. They told their stories.

I felt it was important to hear from everyone, but I was always aware of Kathy.

Kathy quieted down. Every once in a while she'd say, "Ooo, it hurts. It hurts."

Finally, when everybody had told their story, I said to Kathy, "We're in a hospital, and there are doctors in the emergency room. You sound like you're in terrible pain. Would you like to see a doctor?"

And she said, "Yes, I think that's a good idea."

She was wheeled out of the room and taken to the doctor. There was silence again, and deep sadness. We drew our chairs closer together in the circle and we held hands. I went back to the breath, and we started doing conscious breathing.

I go back to the breath because it is so basic and central and calming.

People started swaying while they were seated. This seemed to meet an immediate need.

While the swaying went on, I noticed an autistic, withdrawn posture among the group members, as if this had been too much to deal with. I asked myself: What do I need for myself? What would help my deep sadness and fear about what will happen to Kathy? She was leaving us, and I was watching the process.

While holding hands and swaying backwards and forward, I invited people to bring their thoughts and feelings into the circle.

I wanted to know what was going on with everyone, so I simply asked them. I was facilitating an experience I was also having. I had abdicated a clear role as "teacher" and was just moving through my own feelings in the situation.

We started by swaying in our chairs, and then we stood up and moved the chairs aside. The next thing we did was hold hands. We all sank down onto our knees, and closed up as if we were going inside Kathy's turtle, looking for its kind protection. We stayed there, curled up, for a long time.

I was very careful not to try to over-direct the situation, but to really stay with the fact that I, too, needed to stay where we were for a long time. I would follow the group's initiative.

Finally, one of the men in the group said, "My back hurts."
I said, "What do you want to do?"
He said, "I need to sit up."
I said, "Fine, sit up."

And he put his hands on other people's backs, and they sat up. I said, "Maybe other people would like to have your hand on their backs."

He went around the circle and started putting his hands on people's backs, giving them little massages, as if the turtle shell was being removed. Everybody sat up, and then this man wanted to stand because the sitting position was also uncomfortable for him. He got everybody to stand, and then we started to move in the circle.

I had another question: "What are your thoughts? What is coming up for you? Let's see what images there are to work with. What feelings? I wanted to get all of my clues from the group.

I asked the group these questions. Some people spoke of their love for Kathy and other people said that they became aware of being a tribe, and that they felt a tribal sense at that moment. One talked about being as strong as a fortress and one spoke about feeling the continuity and endlessness of waves rising and falling. People were dealing with what they had come to class with, and this was blending with Kathy's situation.

I heard a lot of different kinds of images. When someone spoke of the fortress I asked her to do a fortress movement. I am interested in the energy of resistance; when there is an opening for strong movement, I usually follow it. This kind of strength can tap into the will to live.

She began stamping. This brought a new dynamic to the room. We went from swaying and being tentative, to finding a pulse which could have been expressing anger, determination, strength, courage, or perseverance. For each person, a movement of that kind of intensity can have a different meaning. We immediately put on some music to reinforce the pulse of the movement. It was Native American music, which isn't moody but straightforward.

I did not want to set up a preconceived mood.

We developed the stomping movement until people began to interact with one another, and we then began to do each other's images in movement. A tribe was formed, and the tribe did a tribal dance. Gradually the movement and the dance brought us into our own collective expression. I had become an active witness and a participant. I stepped out of the role of teacher and let myself be a role model for feeling whatever we were feeling in the moment. By my actions, I was saying, "This is how I feel, and this is how I am expressing it. You can do the same." This gave me the freedom to be present and to communicate what was going on for me. As a result, everyone participated deeply in this class, and the image of the tribe rose organically in our minds, and in our movements.

It was beautiful to see how the group initiated movement to direct themselves. They stopped looking at me for answers. Out of my own sorrow and trust in the group's creative process, I renounced my role as teacher and became part of the group in a different way. I was just me, responding to how I was feeling and how I needed to move. This gave everyone else permission to do the same. All the images they had—fortress, water, tribe—allowed a multi-faceted feeling response to take place. Everybody contributed their own response to Kathy's departure from our group, and together as a group we supported each other. Kathy had found relief from a doctor in emergency. We gave her our drawings as we left. She died a week later.

RE-INVENTING THE FUNERAL

I was teaching my AIDS group, Positive Motion, and Niko came in, absolutely devastated. His best friend had died. He said, "I didn't think I was going to come today, but at the last minute I realized I needed you." He collapsed, and was held while he sobbed.

This was a group I had worked with for a long time. We had shared many experiences with one another, and had a common language in movement. While Niko was crying, I remembered a trust and sensory awareness exercise we had done previously. I was noticing how touch was Niko's most immediate way of connecting. I thought to re-invent this old exercise and put it to another purpose.

I asked the group members to make a linear landscape, a trail, with their bodies. I asked them to sit or stand or lie, while remaining in physical contact with one another. I suggested to Niko that he imagine his life with his friend and begin to move down the landscape of bodies with his eyes closed, while always remaining in physical contact.

I wanted to create an environment that would be nourishing for Niko. I also wanted to create a landscape where his memories and imagination would be involved. Using the sense of touch, and eliminating the sense of sight, often creates new possibilities.

I suggested that as he moved down the line from person to person, he remember another moment with his friend that had been very special for him. Through this touch, and his memories of his friend, he began to mold the way he moved according to the memories he had. The others supported him as he went from one body to the other. Sometimes Niko would lean back to back with somebody. He lay down next to someone who was lying down. Sometimes he wove in and out of people's bodies. This went on for a very long time.

Finally, he came to the end of the trail. I said to him, "Niko, would you like to go outside where the trees are?" He left the group and ran outside. Being inside was very enclosing and soothing, but as soon as he got outside, he just burst open. He opened his eyes and his arms and said, "I release you! And I thank you!"

A deep transformation took place in an hour's time. Movement can change your feelings. I always incorporate the body. Even if I start with an image, I move it through the body. If nothing changes in your body, your feelings will not change.

Brent, another member of the group, said, "It's my birthday today, and I want to do a birthday dance." The group adapted; we went rapidly from Niko's great tragedy to Brent's happy birthday celebration. I suggested to Niko that if he wanted, he could go out into the woods and be by himself, or he could join us.

I wanted to offer him the opportunity to assimilate the experience on his own terms, and not just suddenly jump into something else. Also, being with the sky and the trees seemed like it would be healing for him. The trees could give him a connection to nature, which puts the death experience into a context. It's easier to accept death when you see aspects of it around you in nature.

We did the birthday dance. I asked Brent what he wanted to do, and he said he wanted some music. We picked out something rhythmic and joyful. We made a circle, and he entered into the center. He started dancing, and then brought different people in to dance with him, and directed his own birthday dance. By that time, Niko came back and he joined in the dance of celebration. A ritual of life and death, all in three hours.

As you can see from these four examples, the presence of death always resides in people with life-threatening illness. A facilitator of expressive movement for people in this situation must be willing to work with all the feelings engendered by this reality. Keep your wits and your sense of humor about you, as well as your compassion, and everything you know about the body in motion. Don't forget to feel your feelings while you teach, and that in fact, they are your allies. Observe and listen to your students—their words and bodies will tell you much of what you need to know. If you can't tell from looking or listening, don't be afraid to ask simple questions. How do you feel? What do you need? Where are you now? Trust that movement has the power to transform us, and that our feelings are intimately linked to our physical expression. Access the rich resource of imagery also present in this work. Remember: Always return to the body. Move it, draw it, write about it, share your story.

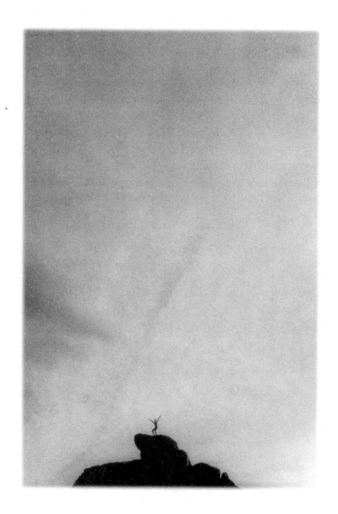

IT'S ABOUT LIVING AND FEELING FULLY THE WHOLE SPECTRUM
FROM JOY TO SADNESS (HOWEVER LONG THAT LASTS) AND DYING
WITH A SENSE OF PEACE (WHENEVER DEATH COMES).

In closing I would like to share with you an excerpt from a letter written to me by my friend Allan Stinson. Allan and I learned many things from one another, and worked together in many different capacities. He studied with me when he was younger and then moved away, and after he contracted HIV, he returned to the Bay Area to make his home. At this time, we began to work together again. He wrote this about the process of healing. I agree with it wholeheartedly.

I am much more at peace, and much healthier, when I listen chiefly to my own body's signals. The real source of my strength and healing is within, and it is important for me to go within, stay there, live there, see from there, meet and make peace with whatever comes through there, and do my reaching out from there. I think that when some of my friends got sick, the fear and the desperation took them a long way out of their bodies in search of a cure. So much so that they almost abandoned their bodies to flee from what was happening inside. Working with movement and visualization is important to me because it helps me turn around, go back down and deep within myself to face, feel, and own my experiences.

As much as I would sometimes wish, I realize I can't send something else down there to do battle in my place: no miracle drug, no surgeon's knife, no megavitamin or micro-diet, no crystal energy, no faith healer's touch, no shaman's prayer, nothing is of any damn value at all unless I am there, fully present with it. I think of healing a little differently than I used to. It's not about living forever or curing the disease. It's about living and feeling fully the whole spectrum from joy to sadness (however long that lasts) and dying with a sense of peace (whenever death comes).

R E S O U R C E   L I S T

B O O K S

IMAGERY IN HEALING, *Jeanne Achterberg, Ph.D.*

RITUALS OF HEALING, *Jeanne Achterberg, Ph.D.*

A GUIDE TO HEALING THROUGH THE HUMAN ENERGY FIELD, *Barbara Brennan*

CANCER AND VITAMIN C, *Ewan Cameron, M.D. and Linus Pauling, Ph.D.*

PERFECT HEALTH, *Deepak Chopra, M.D.*

HEAD FIRST, THE BIOLOGY OF HOPE, *Norman Cousins*

ANATOMY OF AN ILLNESS, *Norman Cousins*

MEANING & MEDICINE - A DOCTOR'S TALE OF BREAKTHROUGH & HEALING, *Larry Dossey, M.D.*

SPONTANEOUS REGRESSIONS OF CANCER, *T.C. Everson and W.H. Cole*

MOVEMENT AWARENESS, *Moshe Feldenkrais*

YOUR PAST LIVES AND THE HEALING PROCESS, *Dr. Adrian Finkelstein*

COMING ALIVE: THE CREATIVE EXPRESSION METHOD, *Daria Halprin-Khalighi, M.A., C.E.T.*

AWAKENING THE SPIRIT: BREATHING KI INTO EVERYDAY LIFE, *Bradford Keeney, Ph.D.*

SPIRITUAL DIMENSIONS OF HEALING, *Stanley Krippner, Ph.D.*

ALTERNATE REALITIES, *Lawrence Leshan, Ph.D.*

CHOICES IN HEALING, *Michael Lerner*

CANCER IN MYTHS AND DREAMS, *Dr. Russell A. Lockhart*

TOWARD A PSYCHOLOGY OF BEING, *Abraham Maslow*

AN INVITATION TO HEALING, *Father Peter McCall and Maryanne Lacy*

RISE AND BE HEALED, *Father Peter McCall and Maryanne Lacy*

I CHOOSE LIFE, *Patricia Norris, Ph.D. and Garrett Porter*

KITCHEN TABLE WISDOM, STORIES THAT HEAL, *Rachel Naomi Remen, M.D.*

CLIENT-CENTERED THERAPY, *Carl R. Rogers*

SEEING WITH THE MINDS EYE, *Mike Samuels and Nancy Samuels*

HOW TO LIVE BETWEEN OFFICE VISITS, *Bernard Siegel, M.D.*

LOVE, MEDICINE AND MIRACLES, *Bernard Siegel, M.D.*

PEACE, LOVE AND HEALING, *Bernard Siegel, M.D.*

GETTING WELL AGAIN, *Stephanie Matthews-Simonton, O. Carl Simonton, and James L. Creighton*

NATURE AS TEACHER AND HEALER - HOW TO AWAKEN YOUR CONNECTION WITH NATURE, *James A. Swan*

ON DREAMS AND DEATH, *Marie-Louise von Franz*

THE SYMBOLIC QUEST, *E.C. Whitmont*

A U D I O T A P E S

Pulse:

AT THE EDGE, *Mickey Hart*

EARTH TRIBE RHYTHMS, THE ULTIMATE DRUM EXPERIENCE, *Brent Lewis*

PULSE, *Brent Lewis*

THE GREAT PLAINS, *Indian Singers and Songs*

RHYTHM HUNTER, *Brent Lewis*

NATIVE GROUND, *One Fine Mama*

TOTEM, *Raven*

BROADCASTING FROM HOME, *Penguin Cafe Orchestra*

Breath:

AMBIENT MUSIC, *Brian Eno*

ANGELS, *Don Campbell*

TANTRIC HARMONICS, *Gyume Tibetan Monks*

THE GYUTO MONKS, *Tibetan Tantric Choir*

DEEP LISTENING, *Pauline Oliveros*

KI, *Kitaro*

SEA SOUNDS, *Didgeridoo*

SKY MIND, *Ray Lynch*

Classical music is also appropriate, but since we are familiar with what is available, it is not listed here.

T A P E S O F S P E C I A L I N T E R E S T

DYING AND DEATH, *Ram Dass*

Write to:

Hanuman Foundation Tape Library

P.M.B. #203

524 San Anselmo Avenue

San Anselmo, CA 94960

1.800.248.1008

FABULOUS JOURNEYS WITHIN: RELAXATION - CHEMOTHERAPY, *Maggie Creighton*

Write to:

Cancer Support and Education Center

1035 Pine Street

Menlo Park, CA 94025

CANCER AS A TURNING POINT, FROM SURVIVING TO THRIVING

Audiotapes by Rachel Remen, J. Bolen, D. Markova, E. Kreidman, C. Auh-Ho-Oh, M. Woodman, S. Campbell, M. Voisard, and V. Boriack.

Write to:

InfoMedia

12800 Garden Grove, Building #F

Garden Grove, CA 92843

For a list of excellent video and audio tape sets by Rachel Naomi Remen, M.D., and Michael Lerner, Ph.D.

Write to:

The Institute for the Study of Health and Illness

A Commonweal Project

P.O. Box 316

Bolinas, CA 94924

VOICES OF HEALING

A documentary telling the stories of five individuals, including Anna Halprin, who face life-threatening illness and find the larger healing of expanded consciousness as they unexpectedly return to health, or go to their dying with humor and grace. By Maureen Redl and Theresa Tollini.

Write to:

Maureen Redl

33 Millwood Road

Mill Valley, CA 94941

Other places to write for cancer resources and support groups:

CENTER FOR ATTITUDINAL HEALING

33 Buchanan

Sausalito, CA

MARIN GENERAL HOSPITAL

250 Bon Air Road

Greenbrae, CA 94914

CANCERPORT
c/o Marin Support
240 Channing Way
San Rafael, CA 94903

B O O K S B Y A N N A H A L P R I N

MOVEMENT RITUAL
Fifteen sequences of floor movements that form a foundation for creative expression, meditation, increased range of movement, flexibility, strength, and physical awareness. The basic movements are done lying on the floor. They are based on anatomical and kinesiological principles. Developed by Anna Halprin in the 1970s, and practiced and expanded upon ever since.

MOVING TOWARD LIFE, FIVE DECADES OF TRANSFORMATIONAL DANCE, *ed. Rachel Kaplan*
Essays, stories, and scores describing the extensive works of Anna Halprin, including the Life/Art Process, Dancers' Workshop, Tamalpa Institute, dance with children, and dance in the environment. Historical document.

CIRCLE THE EARTH MANUAL, *Anna Halprin and Allan Stinson*
Designed for participants of Circle the Earth to enhance their understanding of the philosophy of the dance. Graphic scores, stories, and performance suggestions.

STEPS THEATER COMPANY, *a manual*
Taught by Anna Halprin, documented by Cynthia Imperatore. This is a detailed description of three series of classes from July, 1988 to March, 1989, given to a group of men with HIV and AIDS.

V I D E O S B Y A N N A H A L P R I N & O T H E R S

EXORCISING THE CANCER
A dance performed by Anna Halprin in 1975. She has drawn a life-size self portrait to confront and release her cancer. In this video, you see her dancing her self-portrait. The piece is in three parts: 1) expressing her anger and fear; 2) releasing and dancing her healing; 3) returning to her family and friends.

CIRCLE THE EARTH, DANCING WITH LIFE ON THE LINE, *with Media Arts West*
A documentary of the workshop process from which the healing performance of Circle the Earth developed. This piece was performed by people with HIV/AIDS, cancer, their caregivers, and friends. It is the story of their coming together as a community.

DANCE FOR YOUR LIFE/RITUAL OF LIFE AND DEATH *by Ellison Horne*

A documentary of the classroom work Anna does with people with HIV/AIDS. This is a video of the Steps Theater Company in a workshop setting.

POSITIVE MOTION, *by Andy Abrahams-Wilson*

This video is a collage of seven months of the Steps Theatre Company emotionally charged workshops, culminating in a poignant performance of a work called "Carry Me Home."

THE NATURE SERIES

A collection of five videotapes exploring dance in the environment which show dancers moving with the shapes, rhythms and textures of nature. Intimate and meditative imagery transports us to a place where self and environment merge, to a point of understanding the forces of nature move within us, not outside us.

1. **EMBRACING EARTH,** *by Andy Abrahams-Wilson*
2. **SEASCAPE,** *by Anna Halprin*
3. **CASCADE,** *by Ellison Horne*
4. **A HERO'S JOURNEY,** *by Ellison Horne*
5. **GRIEF AND LOSS,** *by Ellison Horne*

THE POWER OF RITUAL, *an interview with Anna Halprin by Dr. Jeffrey Mishloff*

Originally broadcast as part of the PBS series "Thinking Allowed." Dancing and other ritual activities can allow you to recognize your own inner negativity and to transform its power into healing experience. In this video, Anna draws on her own experience battling cancer to discuss the psychological value of movement and symbolic action.

TOWELLING, DEEP RELAXATION

A video demonstration of how to use a towel for the deep relaxation exercise described in Chapter VIII of this manual. The demonstration is intended to broaden your choices in this exercise, and give ideas on how the towelling movement can be developed.

AUDIO   TAPES   BY   ANNA   HALPRIN

MOVEMENT MEDITATION

A tape designed for people with physical limitations, including the ill and elderly. Movement sequences focus on the breath and the pulse and can be done while seated. The tape explores the breath and the pulse. With music by Pauline Oliveros and Brent Lewis.

MOVEMENT RITUAL LEARNING TAPE

Verbal guidance through each step of Movement Ritual on one side. On the other side, is guided exploration of movement and imagery. See description of Movement Ritual under books. Music by Weldon McCarty.

PHOTO CREDITS

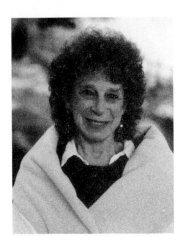

ANNA HALPRIN, PH.D. is a pioneer in the field of dance as a healing art and has been teaching and performing with people challenging cancer, AIDS, and other life threatening illness for the past fifteen years. She is the founder of The San Francisco Dancers' Workshop (1955), an avant-garde performance company, and co-founder of Tamalpa Institute (1978). She has evolved a number of theories for generating a creative process: the most widely known are the Halprin Life/Art Process and the PsychoKinetic Visualization Process. She has received many awards over the years and most recently in 1996 she received the American Dance Festival award for Distinguished Teaching, and in 1997 the prestigious American Dance Festival Award for her Lifetime Achievement in Modern Dance. She teaches in her private Mountain Home Studio in Kentfield, California and tours the United States and abroad. She is the author of *Moving Towards Life*, *Movement Ritual I*, and *Circle the Earth Manual*.

MOUNTAIN HOME STUDIO is Anna Halprin's home studio, located in Marin County, California. Dedicated for over fifty years to the evolution and experimentation of dance and the movement arts, the Mountain Home Studio is nestled among the redwoods of Mount Tamalpais, and adjoined by an outdoor dance deck where students and performers present and create their work. Anna Halprin continues to teach workshops and classes at the Mountain Home Studio throughout the year.

MOUNTAIN HOME STUDIO *15 Ravine Way, Kentfield, CA 94904*
Telephone/Facsimile: 415.461.5362
annahalprin@tamalpa.org
www.tamalpa.org

M I K E   S A M U E L S ,   M . D . has used art and guided imagery with cancer patients for more than 25 years in private medical practice and in consultation. He is also co-founder and director of Art As A Healing Force, a project started in 1990 devoted to making art and healing one. He is the author of fourteen books, including the best selling *Well Body Book*, *Well Baby Book*, *Well Pregnancy Book*, *Seeing With the Mind's Eye*, and *Healing With the Mind's Eye*.

P E G G Y   R O G E R S ,   M . A . ,   M F C C , is Director of Client Services at the Cancer Support and Education Center in Menlo Park, California. She co-facilitates the Self-Empowerment Program, and conducts Facilitator Training Programs. Peggy counsels cancer patients and their families, and gives presentations in imagery and meditation, dealing with cancer, grief and loss. She also leads workshops in communication and the role of expressive therapies in healing.

R A C H E L   K A P L A N is an multi-disciplinary performing artist, writer, and teacher. She tours and teaches in the United States and abroad. She has a unique relationship to Anna Halprin, working both as her personal assistant, and editor of her book projects.

T A M A L P A   I N S T I T U T E is a movement-based expressive arts education organization offering an intensive Training Program, Community Program and a Healing Arts Program. Founded in 1978 by Anna Halprin and Daria Halprin, Tamalpa Institute teaches the Halprin Life/Art Process, an integrative approach to the expressive and therapeutic arts for personal, interpersonal, and social change. The vision of this work is based on the belief that dance and the expressive arts, when connected with the life concerns and issues of the individual, the community, and the environment, have a creative and healing role to play in the lives of all people.

TAMALPA INSTITUTE *Post Office Box No. 794, Kentfield, CA 94914*
Telephone: 415.457.8555 / Facsimile: 415.457.7960
tamalpa@igc.apc.org
www.tamalpa.org

EROS, LOVE & SEXUALITY *by John C. Pierrakos M.D.*

The Forces That Unify Man and Woman

128 pages

In this long-awaited book, Dr. Pierrakos discusses the three great aspects of the life force: eros, love, and sexuality. The free flow of these aspects is our greatest source of pleasure. When we stay open, we experience these aspects as the one life force that generates all activity, all creativity. A student and colleague of Wilhelm Reich, Dr. Pierrakos co-founded Bioenergetics. He later developed Core Energetics, his theraputic work which integrates the higher dimensions of the psyche into our physical existence.

BODY-CENTERED PSYCHOTHERAPY

THE HAKOMI METHOD *by Ron Kurtz*

The Integrated Use of Mindfulness, Nonviolence & the Body

220 pages, illustrations.

A synthesis of philosophies, techniques, and approaches, Hakomi has its own unique artistry, form and organic process. Influences come from general systems theory, incorporating respect for the wisdom of each individual as a living organic system. Hakomi also draws from body-centered psychotherapies such as Reichian work, Bioenergtics, Gestalt, Psychomotor, Feldenkrais, Structural Bodywork, Ericksonian Hypnosis, Focusing, and Neurolinguistic Programing. Hakomi embraces concepts from Buddhism and Taoism, especially gentleness, compassion, mindfulness and going with the grain.

THE HEALING TOUCH *by Malcolm Brown, Ph.D.*

An Introduction to Organismic Psychotherapy

320 pages, 38 illustrations

A moving and meticulous account of Malcolm Brown's journey from Rogerian-style verbal psychotherapist to gifted body psychotherapist. Influenced by C.G. Jung, Abraham Maslow, Erich Neumann, Carl Rogers, D.H. Lawrence, and Wilhelm Reich. Dr. Brown developed his own art and science of body psychotherapy to re-activate the natural mental/spiritual polarities of the psyche and soul. Using powerful case histories as examples, Brown describes the theory, practice and development of his work; techniques to awaken the energy flow and integrate with the main being centers: Eros, Logos, the Spritual Warrior, and the Hara. His unique approach sets a new theraputic guideline with the imaginative and subtle concepts of the embodied soul's psychic dimensions.

CHAKRA BREATHING *Helmut G. Sieczka*

A Pathway to Energy and Harmony

100 pages, illustrations. Supplemental Cassette Tape of Guided Meditations

The breath is the bridge between body and soul. Chakra breathing is meant to activate and harmonize the energy centers of the subtle body. As our lives are increasingly determined by stressful careers and peak performance, the silent and meditative moments become more vital. Chakra breathing enhances emotional and energetic awareness and transformation. Learn to explore and recognize your innate possibilities, and uncover hidden energy potentials.

REIKI *by Baginski & Sharamon*

UNIVERSAL LIFE ENERGY

200 pages, illustrations

The roots of Reiki reach far back into the ancient origins of natural healing. Rediscovered in modern times, Reiki-described as the energy that forms the basis of all life is now widely practiced folk medicine used by practitioners, therapists and healers. Reiki is healing energy in the truest sense of the word, leading to greater individual harmony and attunement to the basic forces of the universe. With the help of specific methods, anyone can learn to use hands to awaken and activate this universal life energy to heal and harmonize energy flow. Based on the authors' experience, this book includes a unique compilation and interpretation of over 200 psychosomatic symptoms and diseases.

A COMPLETE BOOK OF REIKI HEALING *by Müller & Günther*
Heal Yourself, Others, and the World Around You
192 pages, 85 photographs and illustrations
This book outlines the history and practice of Reiki. Photographs and drawings enhance the clear instructions for Reiki hand placement. Brigitte Müller was the first Reiki Master in Europe. She writes about her opening into a new world of healing with the freshness of discovery. Horst Günther experienced Reiki at one of Brigitte's first workshops in Germany, and it changed the course of his life. Together they share a vision of using Reiki universal life energy to help us all to heal ourselves.

LIVING REIKI: TAKATA'S TEACHINGS *Fran Brown*
Stories from the Life of Hawayo Takata
104 pages
In this loving memoir to her teacher, Fran Brown has gathered the colorful stories told by Hawayo Takata during her thirty-five years as the only teaching Reiki Master. The stories create an inspirational panorama of Takata's teachings, filled with the practical and spiritual aspects of a life given to healing.

THE AUTHORITATIVE GUIDE TO GRAPEFRUIT SEED EXTRACT *by Allan Sachs D.C.*
A Breakthrough in Alternative Treatment for Colds, Infections, Candida, Allergies, Herpes, Parasites, and Many Other Ailments
128 pages
Dr. Allan Sachs's innovative treatment of Candida albicans imbalance, food allergies and environmental illness has inspired thousands of patients and a generation of like-minded physicians. Based on his training as a medical reseracher at New York's Downstate Medical Center, and his intense interest in plants, he studied the antimicrobial aspects of certain plant derivatives, especially grapefruit seeds. This handbook provides a background on the therapeutic use of grapefruit seed extract, and details its use for many household, farming and, industrial needs.

THE COSMIC OCTAVE— *Origin of Harmony* by *Cousto*
128 pages, 45 illustrations, numerous tables, 24 page appendix. Specialized planetary tuning forks available.
In this book for astrologers, harmonists, doctors, healers, architects, musicians, or anyone curious about the universe, Hans Cousto demonstrates the direct relationship of astronomical data to ancient and modern measuring systems, the human body, music, and medicine. He writes, "The result is an all-encompassing system of measurement with which it is possible to transpose the movements of the planets into audible rhythms and sounds, and into color. This basic system of measurement clearly demonstrates the harmonic relationship that exists between different kinds of natural phenomena in the fields of astrology, meterology, and microbiology."
Tuning forks calibrated to the tones of the planets, earth, moon and sun, are also available through LifeRhythm.

THE FORGOTTEN POWER OF RHYTHM—*TA KE TI NA* by *R. Flatischler*
160 pages, illustrations. Supplemental CD or Cassette
Rhythm is the central power of our lives, connecting us all. A powerful source of rhythmic knowledge exists in every human being. As we find our way back to this ancient wisdom, we unite with the essence of our life. Reinhard Flatischler presents his brilliant approach to rhythm for both the layman and the professional musician. TA KE TI NA offers the interaction of pulse, breath, voice, walking, and clapping awakening our inherent rhythm in the most direct way-through the body. TA KE TI NA provides first hand knowledge of the rhythmic roots of all cultures, and a new understanding of the many musical voices of our world.

LIFERHYTHM *Connects you with your Core and entire being-guided by Science, Intuition and Love.*
We provide tools for growth, therapy, holistic health and higher education through publications, seminars and workshops.
If you are interested in our forthcoming projects and want to be on our mailing list, send your address to:
P.O. Box 806, Mendocino CA 95460 USA
Telephone: 707. 937.1825 Facsimile: 707. 937.3052
http://www.LifeRhythm.com
books@LifeRhythm.com

Movement has the capacity to take us to the home of the soul, the world

within for which we have no names. Movement reaches our deepest nature,

and dance creatively expresses it. Through dance, we can gain new

insights into the mystery of our inner lives. When brought forth from inside

and forged by the desire to create personal change, dance has the

profound power to heal the body, psyche and soul. Our journey through

illness and health, and the power of dance to illuminate the way,

is a passionate aspect of my life's work.

ANNA HALPRIN